Handbook of Spinal Anaesthesia and Analgesia

Handbook of Spinal Anaesthesia and Analgesia

BENJAMIN G. COVINO
Ph.D., M.D.

Chairman, Department of Anesthesia
Brigham and Women´s Hospital
Professor of Anaesthesia
Harvard Medical School
Boston, Mass., USA

D. BRUCE SCOTT
M.D., F.R.C.P.E., F.R.C. Anaes.

Department of Anaesthetics,
University of Edinburgh,
Edinburgh, Scotland

DONALD H. LAMBERT
Ph.D., M.D.

Department of Anaesthesia
Brigham and Women´s Hospital
Associate Professor of Anesthesia
Harvard Medical School
Boston, Mass., USA

Foreword by
Leroy D. Vandam
M.D.

Coordinator
Lennart Håkansson

Medical drawings
Poul Buckhöj, M.D., h.c.

Anatomical models
Erling Worm Skole, M.D.

W.B SAUNDERS

Preface

Following Koller's description of the topical anaesthetic properties of cocaine in 1884, James Corning, a surgeon in New York City, injected cocaine into the region of the spinal cord of a dog, which resulted in transient hind limb paralysis. Subsequently, Corning administered cocaine spinally into a young patient. However, Corning never mentioned the presence of cerebrospinal fluid and this suggests that the drug may have been injected into the epidural space. In 1899, Augustus Bier, a German surgeon, was the first individual to administer cocaine intrathecally for surgical anaesthesia. Spinal anaesthesia with cocaine was successfully employed in six patients primarily for lower limb orthopaedic procedures. Bier and his colleague, Dr. Hildebrandt, also performed lumbar punctures on each other in order to evaluate the anaesthetic qualities of cocaine administered into the subarachnoid space. The lumbar puncture techniques were rudimentary and resulted in significant loss of cerebrospinal fluid, which led to the first description of post-dural puncture headache.

Following these initial reports, spinal anaesthesia rapidly gained clinical acceptance in Europe and in the United States. It continues to be the most commonly used regional anaesthetic in the United States and it is widely used in the Third World because it is simple, effective and cheap.

After many years of popularity and wide usage, spinal anaesthesia met its greatest challenge when muscle relaxants revolutionized general anaesthesia in the 1940s and 1950s. Indeed in the United Kingdom its use almost stopped completely following the "Wooley and Roe" case in which two patients on the same operating list were permanently paralysed after spinal injections. It is now virtually certain that these tragedies were the result of the antiquated antiseptic measures employed at the time. The use of sterile disposable equipment and sterile packaged ampoules has eliminated such problems, though they must still be taken into account in many parts of the Third World.
In the last decade, there has been a considerable revival in the interest in, and use of, spinal anaesthesia. While many regarded the scientific basis of the technique to have been well established in the first half of the century, modern methods of investigation, especially the double-blind randomized trial, have shown that many of the earlier concepts were flawed. We therefore make no apology for writing this new book on a technique almost 100 years old, in the hope, however vain, that a new broom will remove at least some of the remaining cobwebs.

At the very end of the book we have added a section on the investigation and treatment of neurological complications that may arise following a spinal anaesthetic. Although such conditions are mercifully rare, there is still a tendency for medical staff, other than anaesthesiologists, to jump to conclusions, and such terms as "paraplegia due to spinal anaesthesia" are all too frequently seen in the medical notes. The impact of such a "diagnosis" on the outcome of any legal proceedings against the anaesthesiologist is incalculable. While a patient should have full legal protection against a negligent doctor, doctors should still have the right to defend themselves against the charge of negligence. Perhaps even more important, is that cases involving increased intraspinal pressure can be successfully treated if the diagnosis is made without delay. In any event we are grateful to Dr. Roger Cull, consultant neurologist at the Royal Infirmary, Edinburgh, for his detailed advice on this section.

Throughout the script we have used the International Non-proprietory Names (INN) of the World Health Organization (see p.163) for drug names.

When the preparation of this book was near completion, Ben Covino died suddenly, causing great shock to his family, his colleagues and his many friends. We, his co-authors, feel his absence particularly, as his untiring good humour and wise counsel took us through many hours and days of writing, discussion and rewriting. More importantly we lost a dear and treasured friend. Fortunately Ben's contribution to the book was virtually complete when he died and will be easily discernible to those who knew his style of lecturing and writing. Our own work we offer as a memorial to a great and well-loved man.

Contents

Chapter 1

Anatomical considerations

Vertebral column

The spinal canal runs from the foramen magnum to the sacral hiatus, but the subarachnoid space usually ends at the level of the second sacral vertebra (Fig. 1.1). The spinal cord usually ends at the upper border of the second lumbar vertebra though this can vary between T12 and L3. It is therefore safest to enter the subarachnoid space below L2. However, the subarachnoid space can be entered at higher levels if there are special indications for doing so.

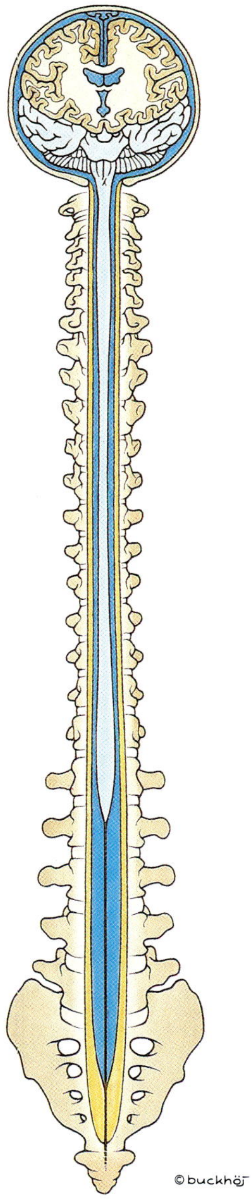

Fig. 1.1.

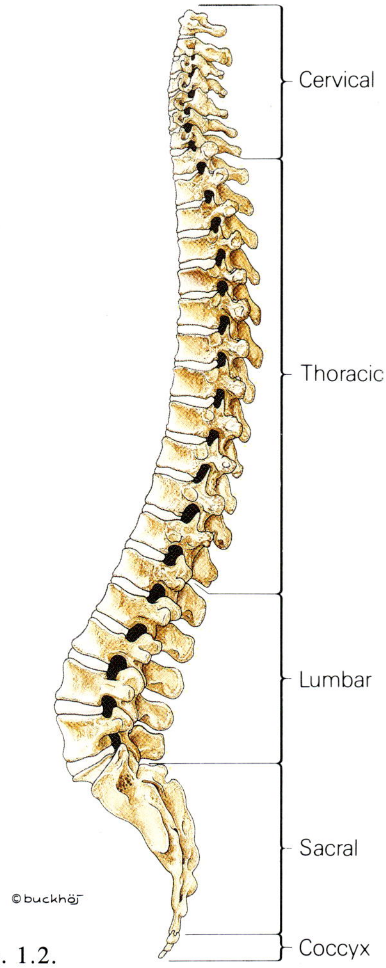

Fig. 1.2.

Vertebrae

The spinal column is made up of 7 cervical, 12 thoracic and 5 lumbar vertebrae, with the sacrum and coccyx inferiorly (Fig. 1.2). They are held together by the vertebral ligaments. Each vertebra has a ring of bone attached posteriorly to its body, thus forming the spinal canal running from the foramen magnum to the coccyx. Adjacent vertebral bodies in the cervical, thoracic and lumbar regions are separated by the intervertebral discs.

Though all the vertebrae have a common structure (Fig. 1.3), they vary in shape and size according to their position and function. The cervical vertebrae, having the least weight bearing and the maximum amount of movement, are relatively small compared with the large robust vertebrae in the lumbar region (Fig. 1.4).

A vertebra is made up of a vertebral body behind which is a bony arch (Fig. 1.3). The arch consists of two pedicles anteriorly and two laminae posteriorly. At the junction of pedicles and laminae are the transverse processes. Where the laminae meet is the spinous process.

The spinous processes vary in regard to their angulation. In the cervical, upper and lower thoracic, and lumbar regions they are almost horizontal. In the mid-thoracic region, however, the spinous processes are directed caudally and this angulation becomes maximal between T3 and T7 (Fig. 1.2).

Fig. 1.4. Oblique views of a thoracic and a lumbar vertebra.

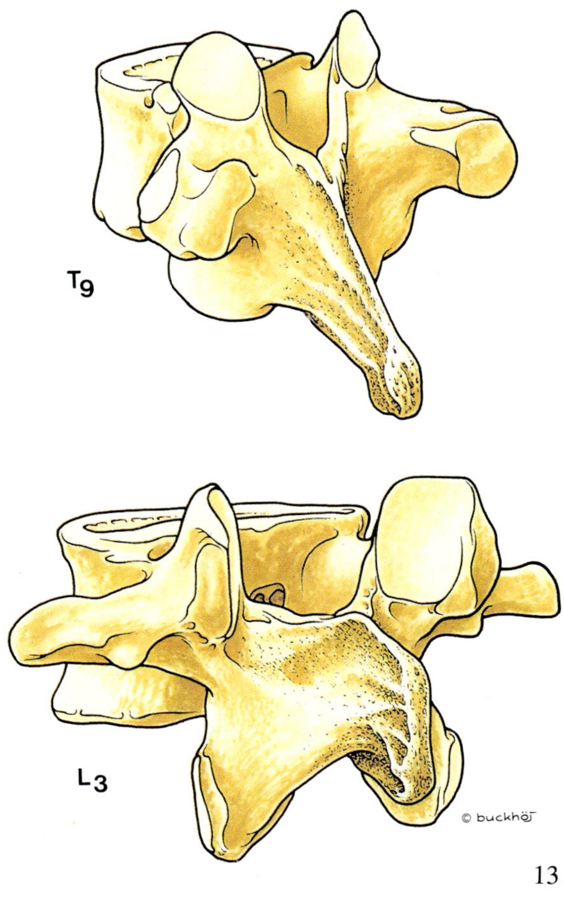

Fig. 1.3. Typical thoracic vertebra.

1. Spinous process
2. Lamina
3. Vertebral foramen (spinal canal)
4. Transverse process
5. Superior articular process
6. Pedicle
7. Vertebral body

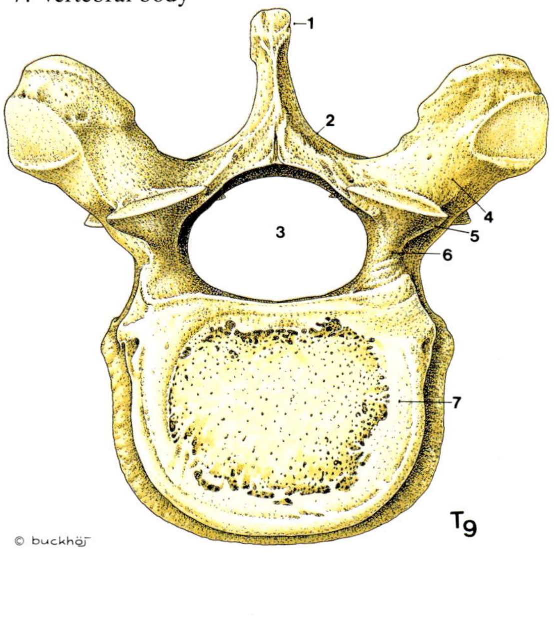

The sacrum is formed by the fusion of the 5 sacral vertebrae inside which the spinal canal continues downwards to end at the sacral hiatus, which is a gap in the fifth sacral vertebra due to the absence of its laminae (Figs. 1.5a and b). Occasionally the laminae of S4 and even S3 are also absent, causing an abnormally large hiatus. The coccyx is attached to the sacrum inferiorly.

Figs. 1.5. a: Posterior view and b: sagittal section of the sacrum and coccyx.

1. S4
2. Sacral hiatus
3. Sacrococcygeus ligament

a

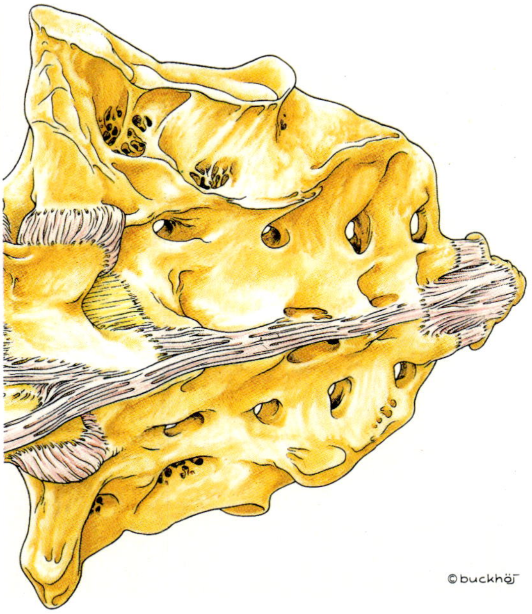

b

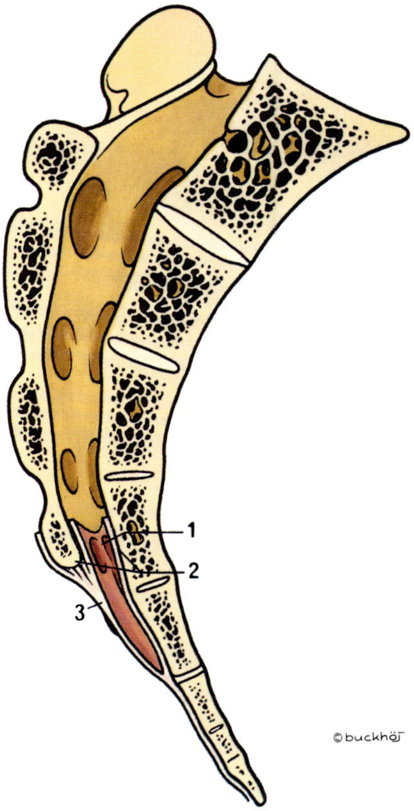

Spinal ligaments

Adjacent vertebrae are held together posteriorly by short tough ligaments and it is through these ligaments that a needle must pass to reach the spinal canal. The laminae of the vertebrae are connected by the ligamentum flavum while the spinous processes are connected by the interspinous ligament. The supraspinous ligament runs superficial to the tips of the spinous processes. Anteriorly the bodies of the vertebrae are separated by the intervertebral discs and the anterior longitudinal ligament runs from the skull to the sacrum with firm attachments to the discs and the adjacent margins of the vertebral bodies. The posterior longitudinal ligament connects the posterior aspects of the vertebral bodies and forms the anterior wall of the vertebral canal (Fig. 1.6).

The pedicles are not connected by ligaments, and it is through the resulting aperture, the intervertebral foramen, that the spinal nerves leave the spinal canal.

To insert a needle into the spinal canal between two vertebrae in the midline, it must traverse the supraspinous and interspinous ligaments before reaching the ligamentum flavum, the last barrier to the canal itself (Fig. 1.7). With a paramedian approach the needle will miss the supraspinous and interspinous ligaments and the only ligament to be penetrated is the ligamentum flavum.

Fig. 1.6. Cross-section of a lumbar vertebra showing the attachment of the spinal ligaments.

1. Supraspinous ligament
2. Interspinous ligament
3. Ligamentum flavum
4. Posterior longitudinal ligament
5. Anterior longitudinal ligament

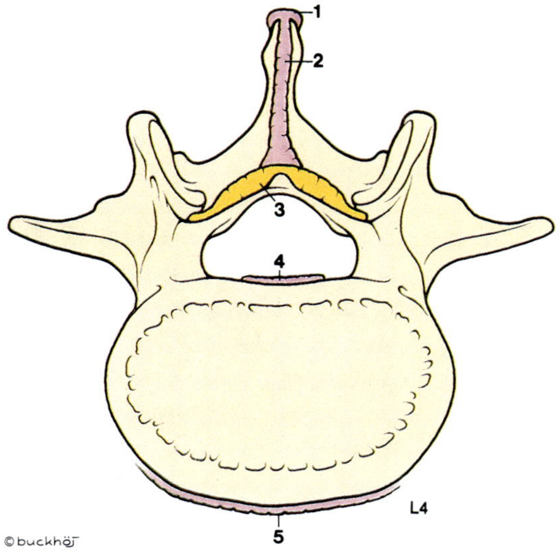

Fig. 1.7. Sagittal section through the second and third lumbar vertebrae showing the ligaments attached to adjacent laminae and spinous processes.

1. Supraspinous ligament
2. Interspinous ligament
3. Ligamentum flavum

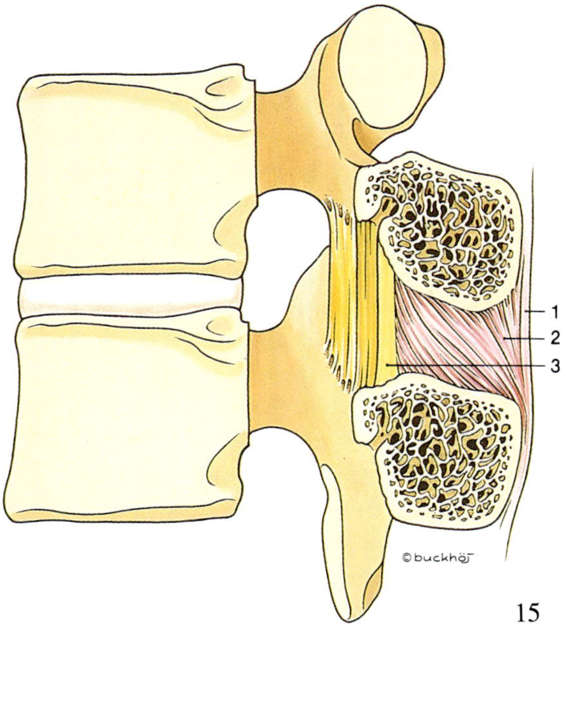

The ligamentum flavum is tougher than the other ligaments and it is usually easy to identify by its increased resistance to the needle. It is thinnest in the midline, getting thicker laterally (Fig. 1.8). Its function is to hold adjacent laminae firmly together and it forms, together with the laminae, the posterior wall of the spinal canal.

In some subjects, the ligamentum flavum is a continuous band with no division in the midline. In others there is such a division, through which blood vessels pass into and out of the spinal canal. These divisions account for the minimal resistance to the advancing needle occasionally encountered when performing lumbar puncture. Both types of ligament can be seen at different intervertebral spaces in the same subject.

Fig. 1.8. Ligamentum flavum showing thin area in the midline.

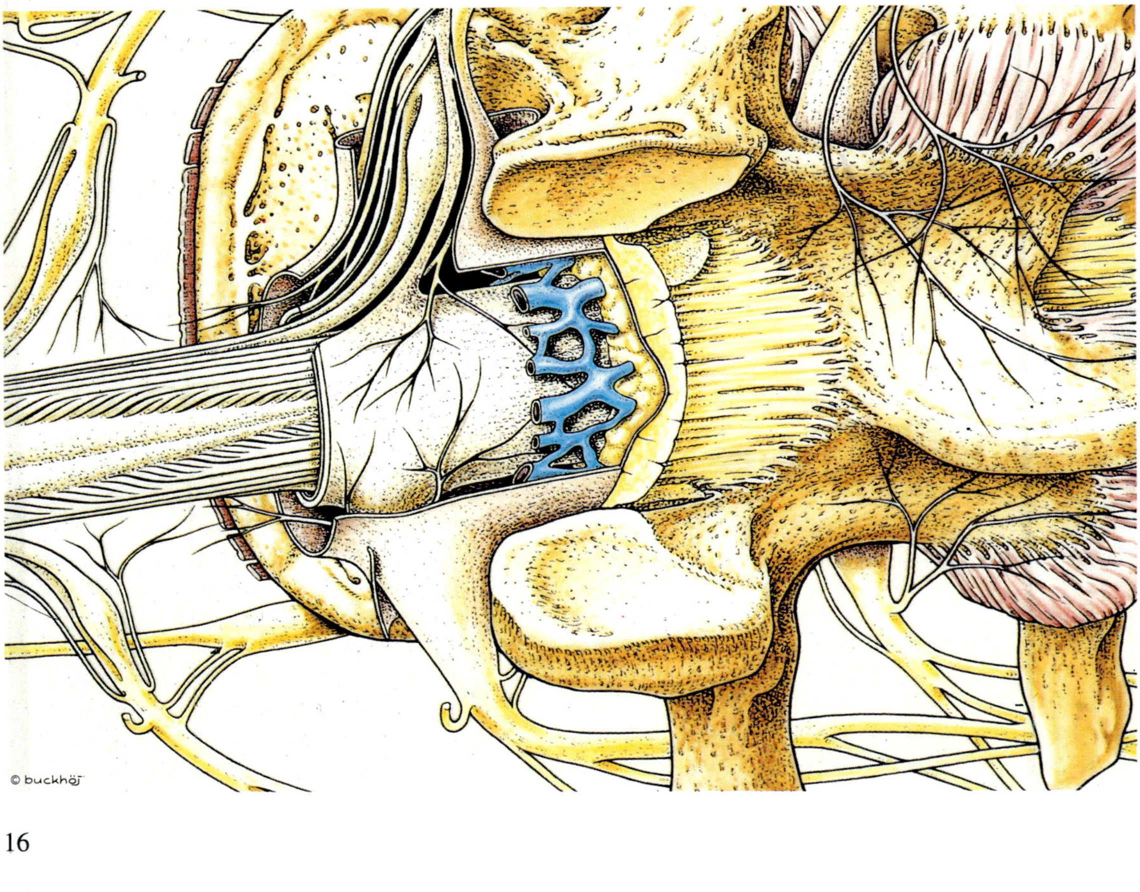

Spinal meninges

Within the spinal canal there are three sleeves of connective tissues, the dura mater, the arachnoid mater and the pia mater, which cover and protect the spinal cord. They form three spaces, the epidural space, the subdural space and the subarachnoid space (Fig. 1.9).

The epidural space is that part of the spinal canal between its outer wall and the dura mater. It is only a potential space. It contains:

a. fat,
b. he spinal nerves as they leave the spinal canal through the intervertebral foramina,
c. blood vessels supplying the vertebrae and the spinal cord.

Fig. 1.9. Cross-section of the spinal canal in the thoracic region showing the spinal ligaments and the contents of the dural sac.

1. Posterior longitudinal ligament
2. Periosteum
3. Nerve root
4. Subarachnoid space
5. Epidural space
6. Pia mater
7. Arachnoid mater
8. Subdural space
9. Subarachnoid septum
10. Dura mater (inner layer)
11. Dura mater (outer layer)
12. Ligamentum flavum
13. Ligamentum denticulatum
14. Dorsal nerve root
15. Ventral nerve root
16. Dorsal root ganglion
17. Spinal nerve

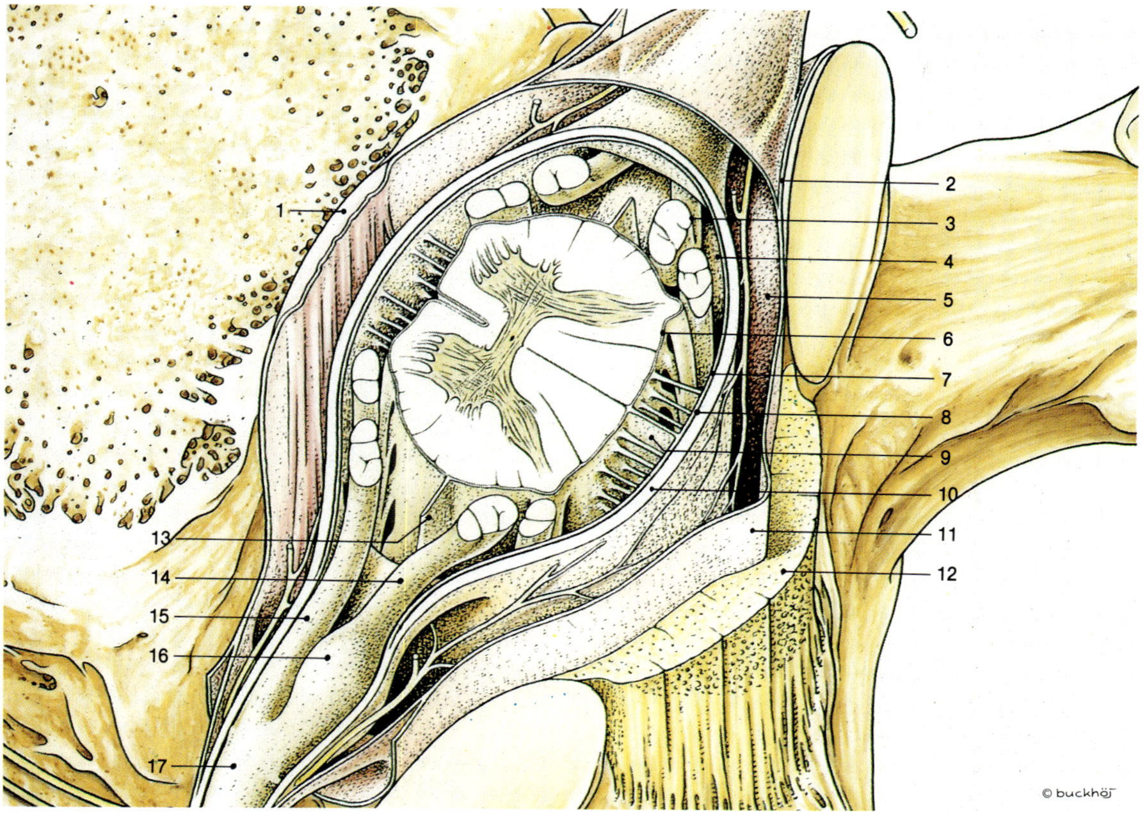

As the dura mater is attached to the foramen magnum and the first and second cervical vertebrae, fluid injected into the epidural space cannot ascend into the cranium.

A continuous sheet of connective tissue covers the wall of the spinal canal and is usually referred to as "periosteum". However, it not only covers the bony wall but also the ligaments joining adjacent vertebrae and the intervertebral discs. Unlike true periosteum, it can be lifted off the bone relatively easily. Some anatomy textbooks refer to it as the "outer layer" of the dura mater. Thin irregular bands of tissue run between these two layers (Figs. 1.9 and 10).

On the inner side of the dura mater is the arachnoid mater, which is closely applied but not physically attached to the dura. The potential space between the dura and arachnoid mater is the subdural space (Figs. 1.9 and 10).

The subarachnoid space lies between the arachnoid and the pia mater. It contains the spinal cord, the nerve roots and the cerebrospinal fluid (Figs. 1.9 and 10). The spinal and cranial subarachnoid spaces communicate freely through the foramen magnum. Between the pia and arachnoid mater run numerous fine strands (trabeculae). In addition there are two fibrous bands which suspend the spinal cord in a central position within the spinal canal, the ligamentum denticulatum and the subarachnoid septum (Fig 1:11).

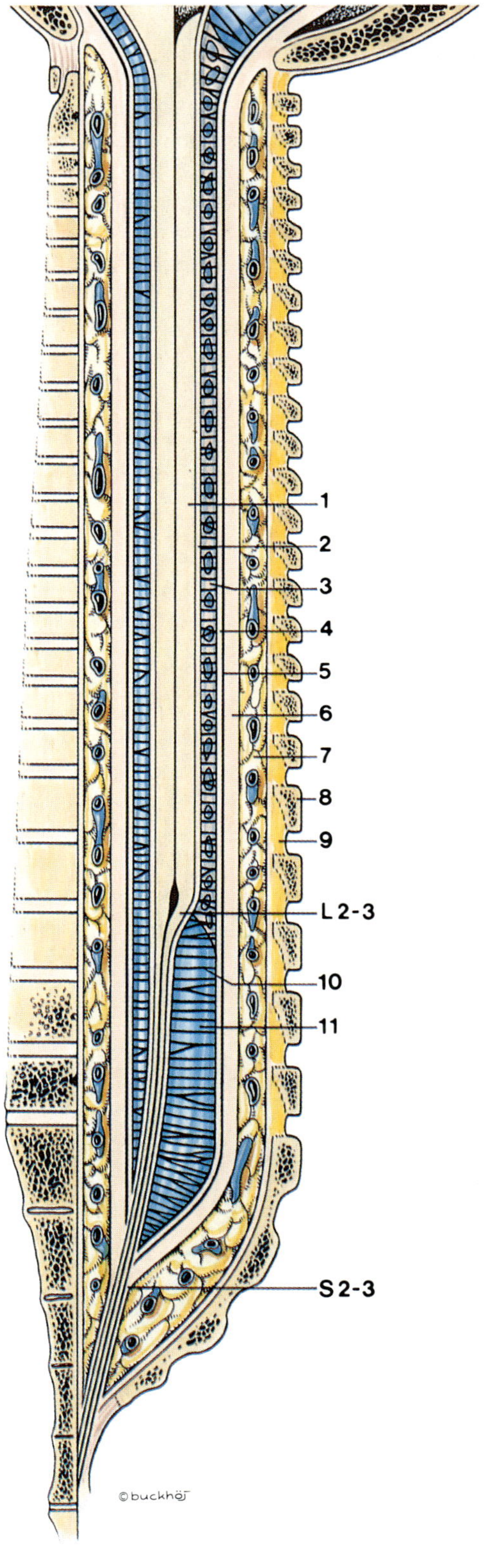

Fig. 1.10. Schematic diagram showing the levels at which the epidural space, the subarachnoid space and the spinal cord terminate.

1. Spinal cord
2. Pia mater
3. Subarachnoid septum
4. Arachnoid mater
5. Subdural space
6. Dura mater
7. Epidural space
8. Vertebra
9. Ligamentum flavum
10. Trabecula
11. Subarachnoid space

The ligamentum denticulatum, which is found on each side of the spinal cord, is continuous with the pia mater between each set of anterior and posterior nerve roots. It has triangular projections reaching to the arachnoid mater (Fig. 1.11). The subarachnoid septum joins the pia and arachnoid in the median plane posteriorly (Fig. 1.11). It is not a complete septum, being cribriform, but may offer some barrier to the free spread of injected solutions, particularly in the thoracic region.

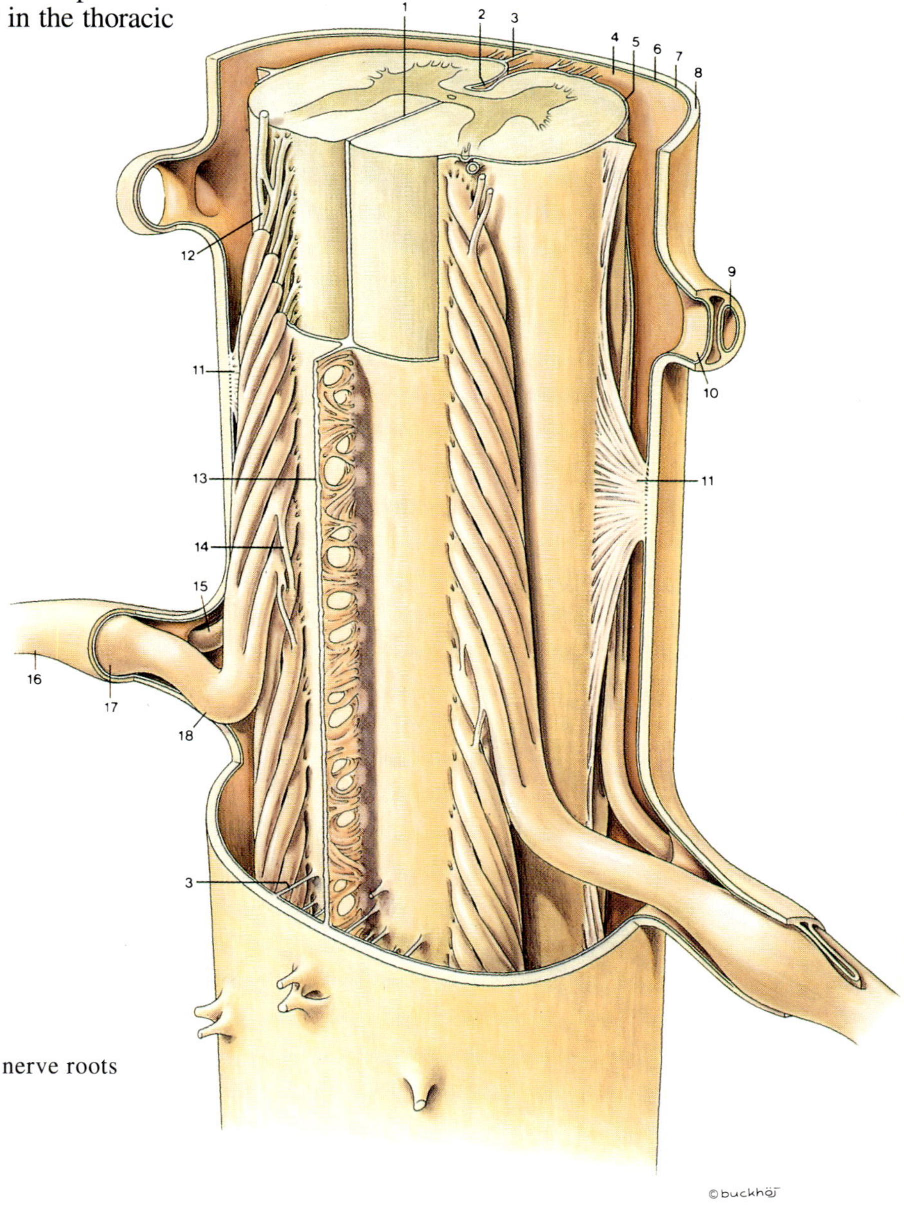

Fig. 1.11.

1. Posterior median septum
2. Anterior median fissure
3. Trabecula
4. Subarachnoid space
5. Pia mater
6. Arachnoid mater
7. Subdural space
8. Dura mater
9. Space for ventral nerve root
10. Space for dorsal nerve root
11. Ligamentum denticulatum
12. Rootlets
13. Subarachnoid septum
14. Nerve fibres interconnecting nerve roots of adjacent segments
15. Ventral nerve root
16. Spinal nerve T 10
17. Dorsal root ganglion
18. Dorsal nerve root

Dura mater

The dura mater is a sheet of firm connective tissue made up of collagen, elastic fibres and ground substance. It varies considerably in thickness, even in the same individual.

Microscopically it is seen to be arranged in concentric lamellae which branch irregularly.[1] Electron microscopy shows that the collagen fibres interlace in a wavy irregular manner and do not have a marked directional alignment. The elastic fibres, on the other hand, are directed both longitudinally and transversely. This arrangement of the fibres (Fig. 1.12) indicates that a dural hole caused by a spinal needle tip directed longitudinally would gape less during spinal flexion, compared to a bevel directed transversely.

Viewed with an epiduroscope, the dura can be seen to indent several millimetres without penetration when impinged upon by a large and relatively blunt epidural needle (Fig. 1.13).

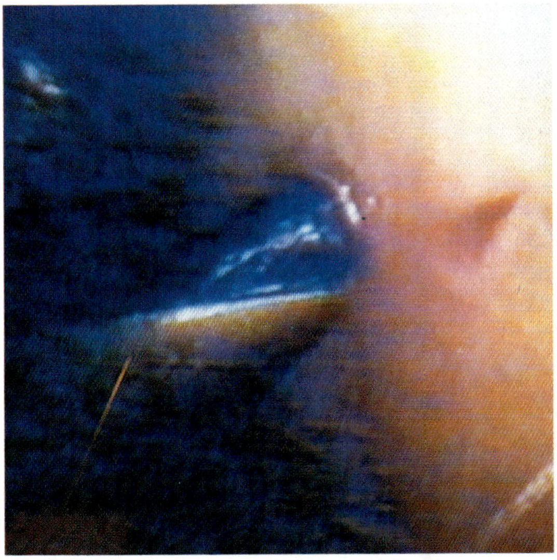

Fig. 1.13. Epiduroscopic view of the dura mater and epidural space. (Courtesy of Dr. N. Rawal)

Fig. 1.12. Electron micrograph of posterior lumbar dura mater (cylinder and plane indicate how the tangential longitudinal section was taken from the specimen). The arrangement of the collagen was very variable. The direction of the elastic fibres (arrows) was consistent in all sections and planes. Courtesy of Dr. B. Raymond Fink

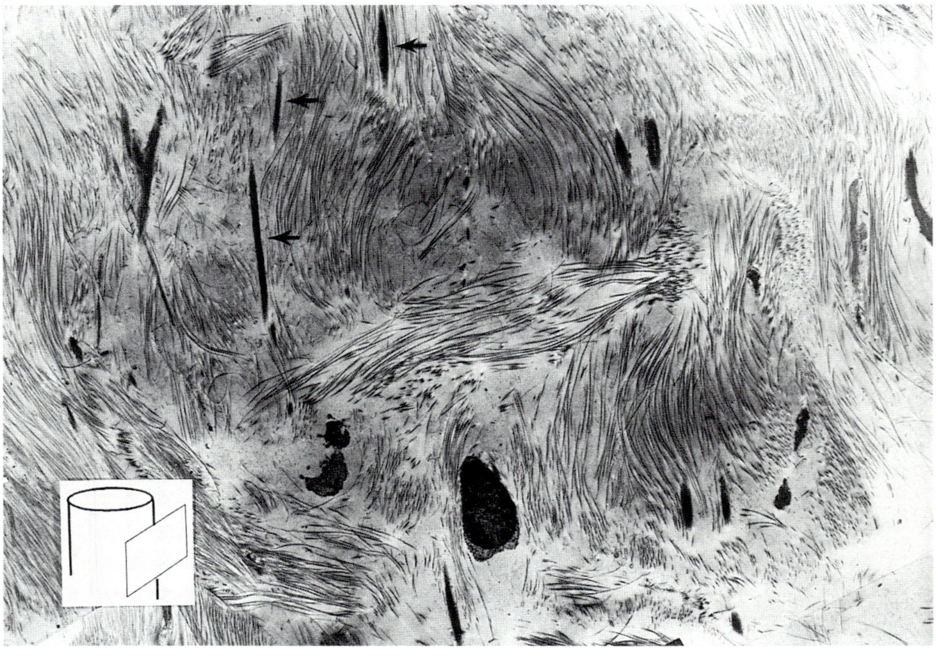

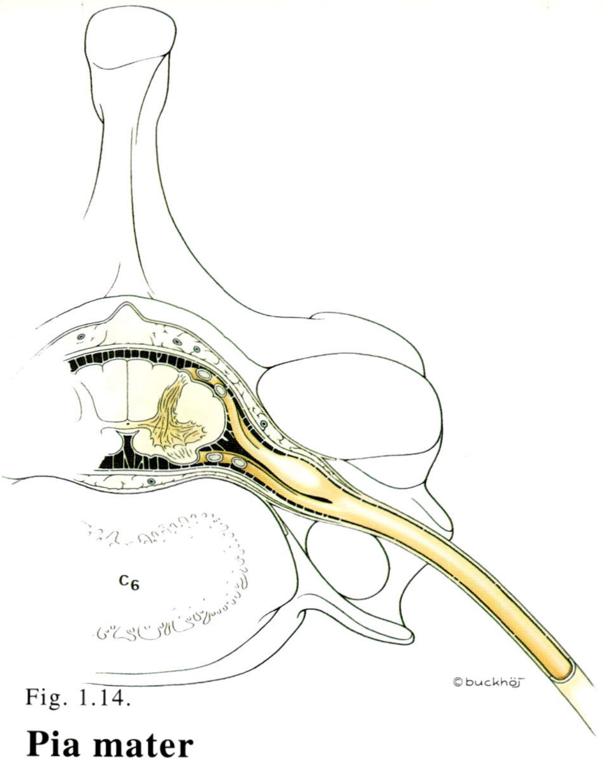

Fig. 1.14.

Pia mater

The pia mater closely invests the spinal cord and its blood vessels, and is continuous with the cerebral pia mater (Fig. 1.15). It consists of two layers; the inner one is in intimate contact with the glial cells, and cannot be stripped from the spinal cord. The blood vessels which run along the spinal nerve roots and the spinal cord stand out clearly and are covered with pia mater. Microscopically this covering extends to the commencement of the capillaries.

Fig. 1.15. Photograph of the spinal cord covered by the pia mater.

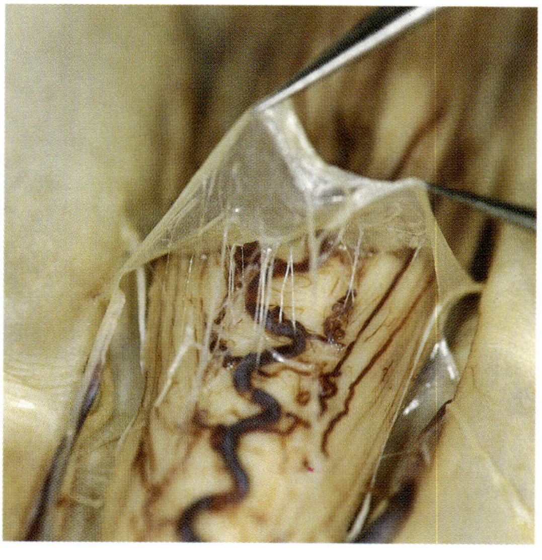

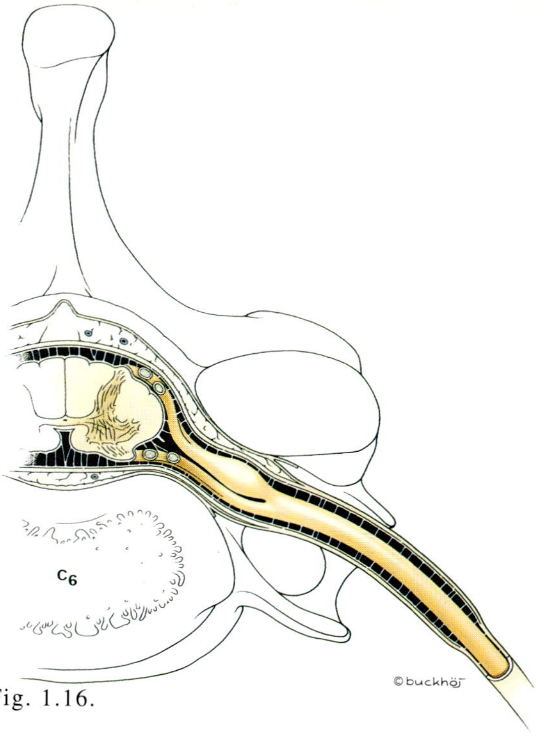

Fig. 1.16.

The three meninges also extend laterally to invest first the spinal nerve roots and then the mixed spinal nerves. The pia, arachnoid and dura mater thus form the connective tissue of nerves, as the endoneurium, perineurium and epineurium. The subarachnoid space also extends laterally along the nerve roots and mixed nerves for a short distance (Fig. 1.14). These dural cuffs usually end at the intervertebral foramina, but occasionally they extend a centimetre or more along the mixed spinal nerves (Fig. 1.16).

The spinal cord

The spinal cord is continuous with the medulla oblongata of the brain and runs from the level of the foramen magnum to the upper border of the second lumbar vertebra, an average length of 45 cm. Though it tapers from above to below, it has two enlargements, the cervical and the lumbar, which correspond to the innervation of the upper and lower limbs. Its tip is attached to the filum terminale, a band of connective tissue which descends to end at the coccyx (Fig. 1.17). In a minority of subjects the spinal cord ends below L2, occasionally reaching the lower border of L3 (Fig. 1.17).

Along the anterior surface is the anterior median fissure, which on cross-section is seen to extend to a depth of 3 mm into the cord (Fig. 1.18). This fissure contains pia mater and blood vessels supplying the central region of the spinal cord (Fig. 1.20). Posteriorly is a less marked indentation, the posterior median sulcus. The posterior median septum, a sheet of neuroglia, extends almost to the central canal, effectively dividing the right and left side of the white matter of the cord posteriorly. Anteriorly the median fissure does not reach the grey matter and nerve fibres do cross the midline in the white matter dorsal to the fissure.

On each side of the spinal cord are the posterolateral sulci along which the dorsal spinal roots enter the cord.

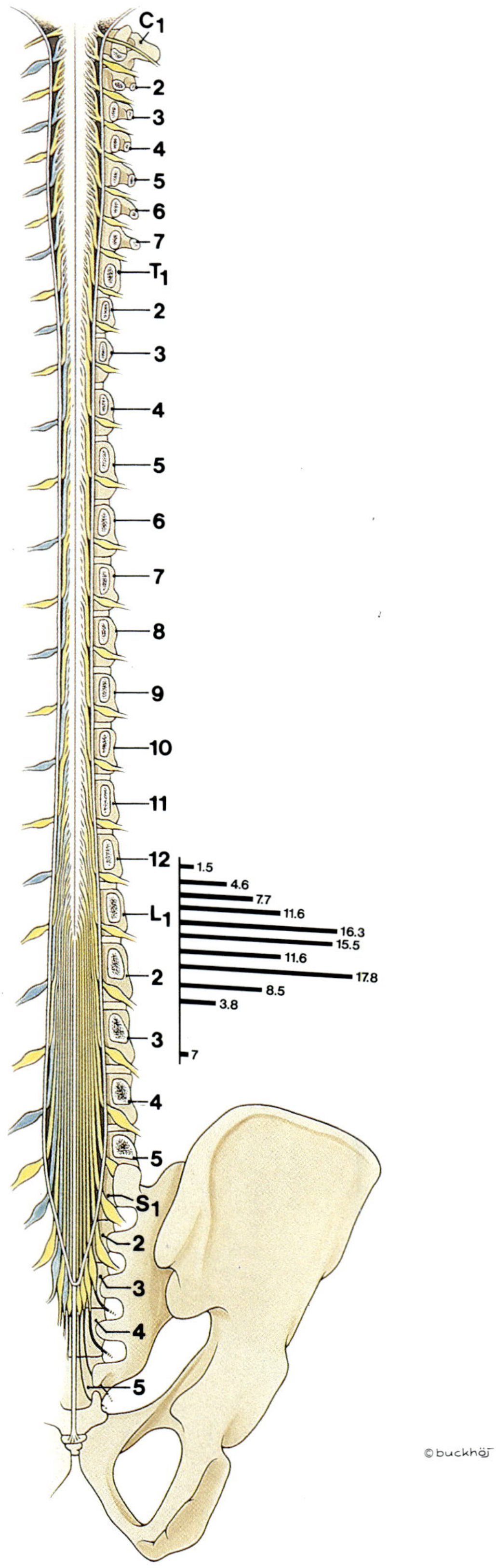

Fig. 1.17. The spinal cord, spinal nerves and the filum terminale. The horizontal bars indicate the percentage of specimens that ended at the level shown. (After Reimann and Anson[2])

Fig. 1.18. Cross-section of the spinal canal at T11.

1. Ligamentum denticulatum
2. Posterior median septum
3. Anterior median fissure
4. Posterior longitudinal ligament
5. Pia mater
6. Dura mater
7. Subdural space
8. Arachnoid mater
9. Subarachnoid space
10. Ventral nerve root
11. Dorsal nerve root
12. Dorsal root ganglion
13. Anterior meningeal branch to epidural and subarachnoid space
14. Epinerium (continuation of dura mater)
15. White ramus communicans
16. Gray ramus communicans
17. Spinal nerve T 11
18. Intercostal nerve (ventral ramus)
19. Perineurium (continuation of arachnoid mater)
20. Dorsal ramus of spinal nerve
21. Posterior meningeal branch to epidural and subarachnoid space
22. Dorsal root of T 11
23. Dorsal root of T 12
24. Dorsal root of L1
25. Dorsal root of L2
26. Dorsal root of L3
27. Trabecula
28. Subarachnoid septum

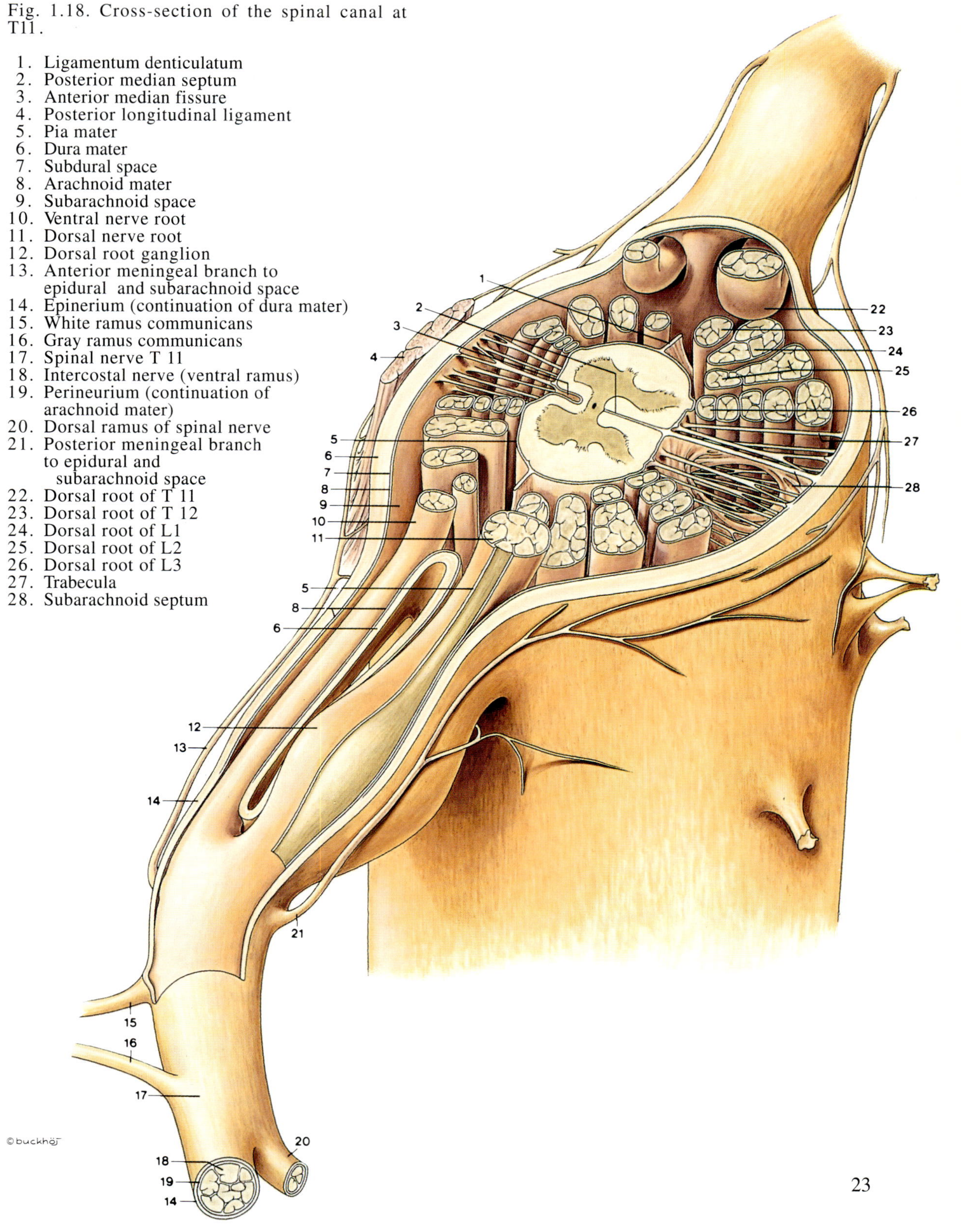

Blood supply

The spinal cord is supplied with blood from the spinal branches of the vertebral, deep cervical, intercostal and lumbar arteries (Fig. 1.19). These spinal branches divide into anterior and posterior radicular arteries which travel along the nerve roots to reach the cord, and divide to form a plexus of arteries in the pia mater (Fig. 1.20).

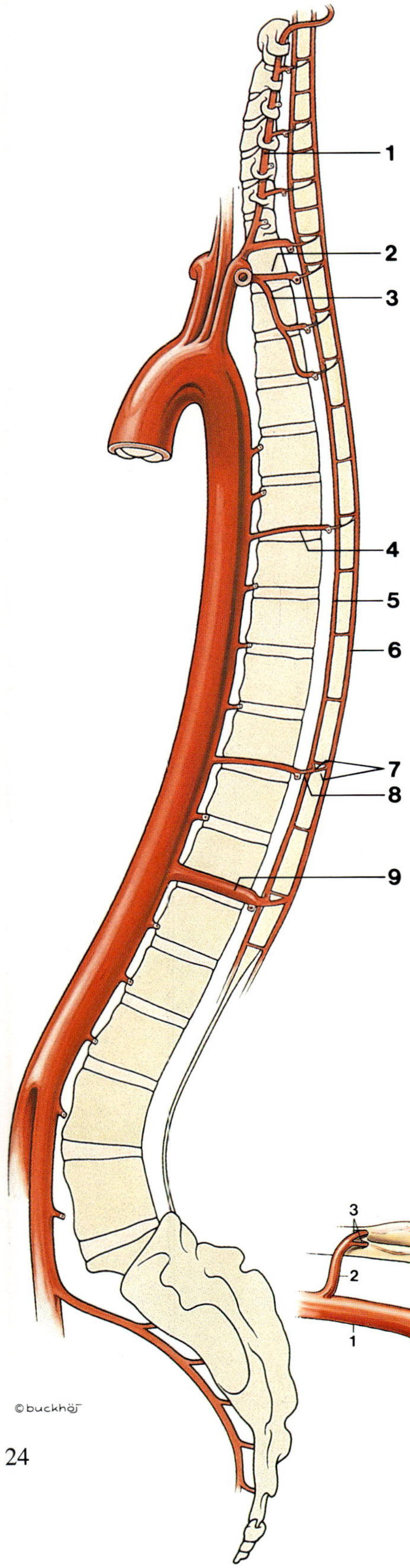

Fig. 1.19. Arterial supply to the spinal cord.

1. Vertebral artery
2. Deep cervical artery
3. Superior intercostal artery
4. Intercostal artery
5. Anterior spinal artery
6. Posterior spinal artery
7. Anterior and posterior radicular arteries
8. Spinal branch of intercostal artery
9. Artery of Adamkiewicz

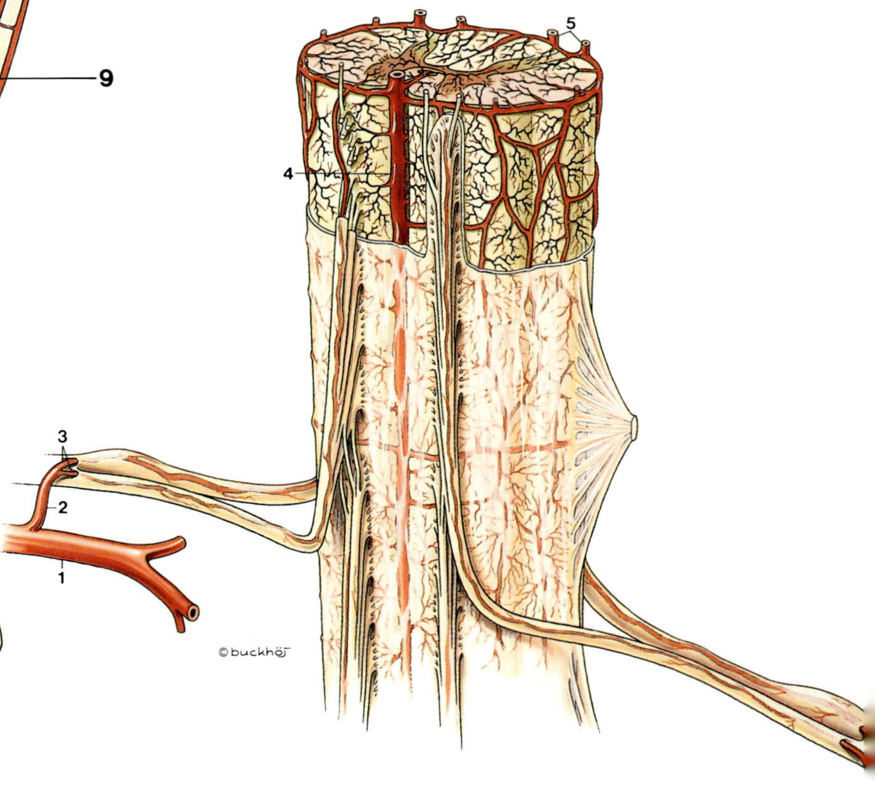

Fig. 1.20. Arterial supply to the spinal cord, anterior view.

1. Intercostal artery
2. Spinal branch of the intercostal artery
3. Anterior and posterior radicular arteries
4. Anterior spinal artery
5. Posterior spinal arteries

Most of the anterior radicular branches end in the anterior nerve roots, but a variable number send superior and inferior branches which anastomose with similar arteries above and below, thus forming a single longitudinal vessel along the median sulcus of the cord, i.e. the anterior spinal artery (Fig. 1.20). Usually one radicular artery is much larger than the rest and is responsible for the major part of the blood supply to the lower two-thirds of the cord. This is known as the arteria radicularis magna or the artery of Adamkiewicz, and it arises in either the lower thoracic or the upper lumbar region. It is more common on the left side than on the right (Fig. 1.19).

Posterior radicular arteries run along the posterior roots and by anastomoses above and below give rise to two posterior spinal arteries on either side of the attachment of the dorsal roots (Figs. 1.20 and 21). The anterior spinal artery supplies the anterior two-thirds of the cord and the posterior spinal arteries supply the remainder, with a contribution from the plexus in the pia mater supplied by branches of the radicular arteries. There are no arterial anastomoses within the cord, though there is some overlap of distribution.

Fig. 1.21.A. Blood supply to the spinal cord, posterior view. B. Cross-section of the spinal cord showing the blood supply.

1. Spinal branch of intercostal artery
2. Anterior and posterior radicular arteries
3. Posterior spinal arteries
4. Anterior spinal artery

1. Anterior spinal artery
2. Anterior spinal vein
3. Posterior spinal vein
4. Posterior spinal artery radicular
5. Anterior and posterior.arteries
6. Spinal branch of intercostal artery

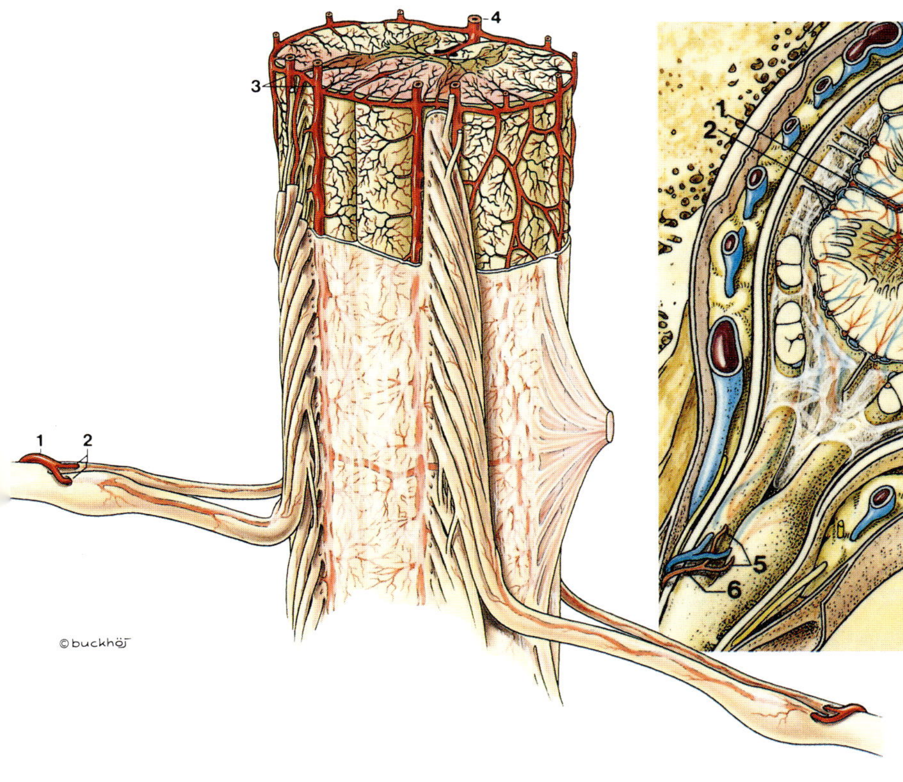

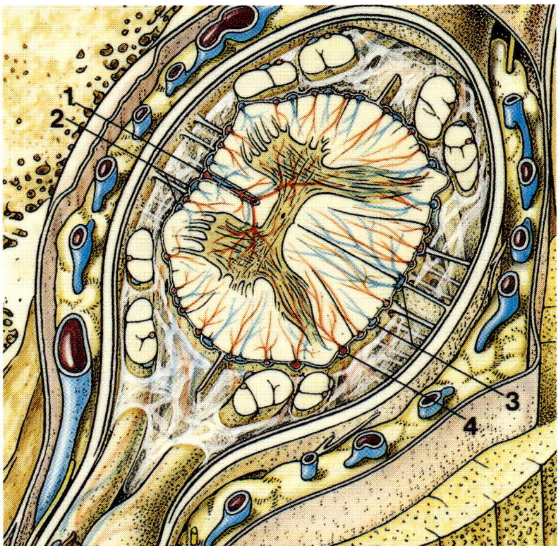

Blood from the spinal cord drains into a tortuous venous plexus within the pia mater (Fig. 1.14), which contains six longitudinal vessels. These connect with the internal vertebral plexus in the epidural space, which is drained via the intervertebral veins into the azygos and hemiazygos venous systems (Fig. 1.22).

Blood from the vertebrae drains into both the internal and the external vertebral plexuses. To reach the external plexus the veins must traverse the ligamenta flava or leave the vertebrae directly (Fig. 1.23).

Fig. 1.22. Cross-section of the thoracic spine showing the venous drainage of the vertebrae and spinal cord.

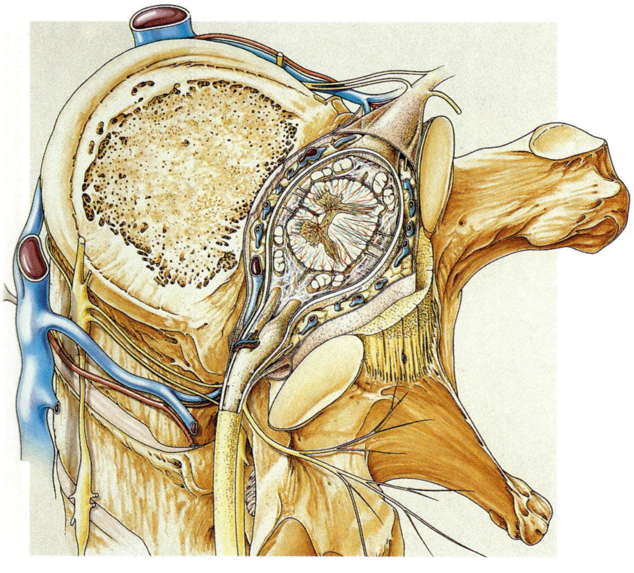

Fig. 1.23. Venous drainage of the vertebrae

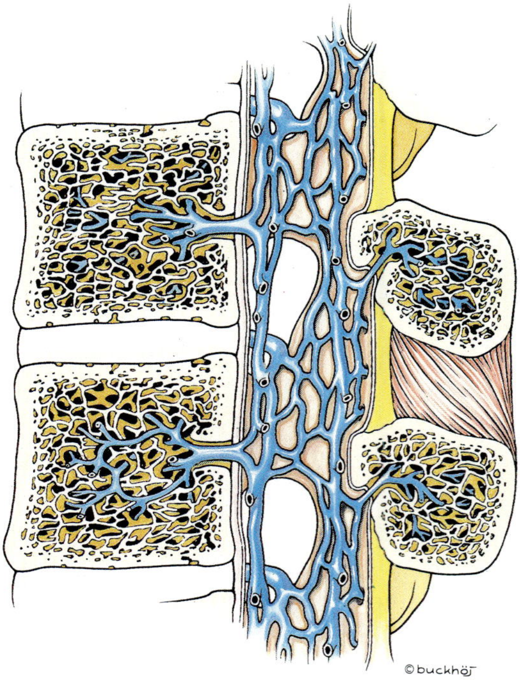

Spinal nerves

There are 31 pairs of spinal nerves, 8 cervical, 12 thoracic, 5 lumbar, 5 sacral and 1 coccygeal (Fig. 1.24).

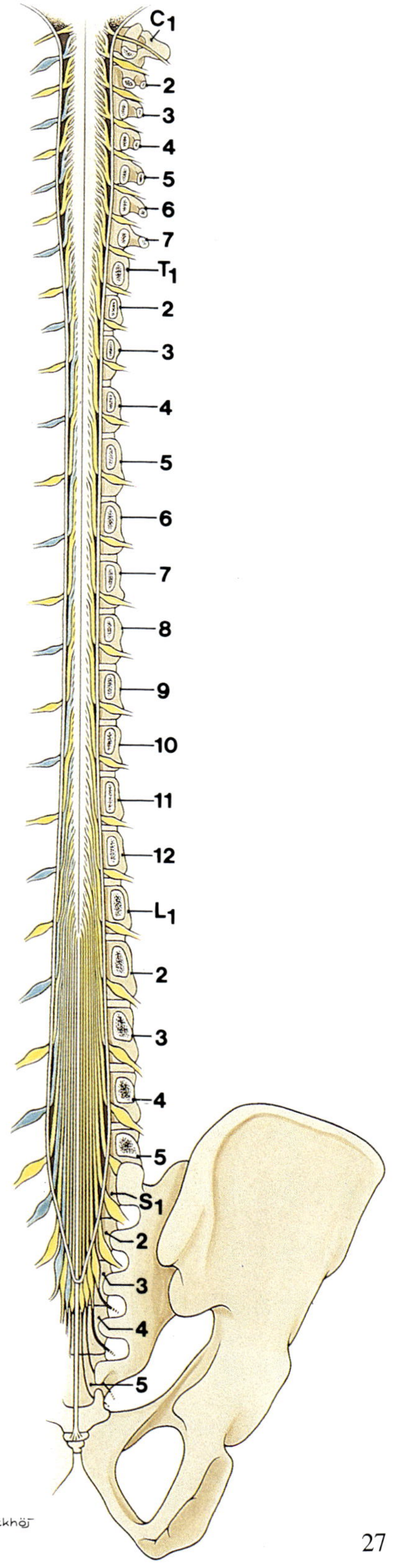

Fig. 1.24. The relation of the spinal column to the nerve root origins from the spinal cord.

Each nerve is formed by the union of a ventral and a dorsal root. Each root is made up of several rootlets which connect to the spinal cord (Fig. 1.25). Laterally each ventral and dorsal root pierces the arachnoid and dura separately before uniting at or near the intervertebral foramen to form the mixed spinal nerve.

The dorsal roots each have an enlargement, the dorsal root ganglion, which contains the nerve cells of the somatic and autonomic sensory nerves.The dorsal root ganglia are found at a variable distance from the spinal cord, and are not uncommonly located lateral to the point where the two roots join.

Fig. 1.25. The dorsal rootlets and roots of a spinal nerve.

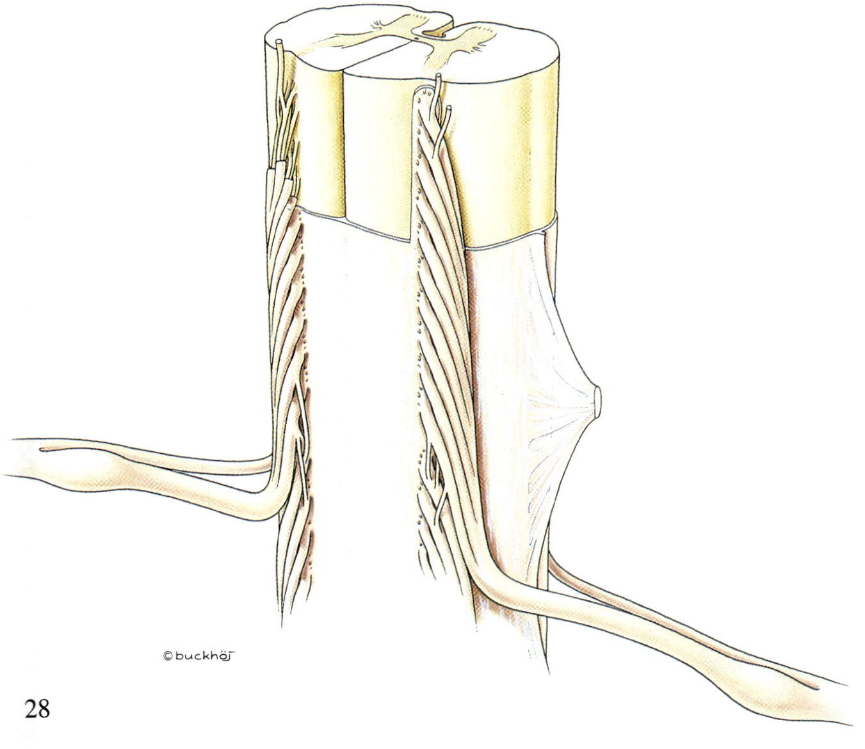

After the two roots join, both sensory and motor nerve fibres mix, according to their eventual destination. They are organised into fasciculi each containing a variable number of nerve fibres.

Each fibre is surrounded by connective tissue, the endoneurium, and each fasciculus by the perineurium. Surrounding a collection of fasciculi, i.e. a mixed nerve, is the epineurium (Fig. 1.26). These connective tissue components of the nerves derive from the meninges (p. 21).

Fig. 1.26.

1. Epineurium
2. Fat cell
3. Fasciculus
4. Perineurium
5. Endoneurium
6. Schwann cell sheath (myelin sheath)
7. Axon
8. Nucleus of Schwann cell
9. Myelinated nerve fibre

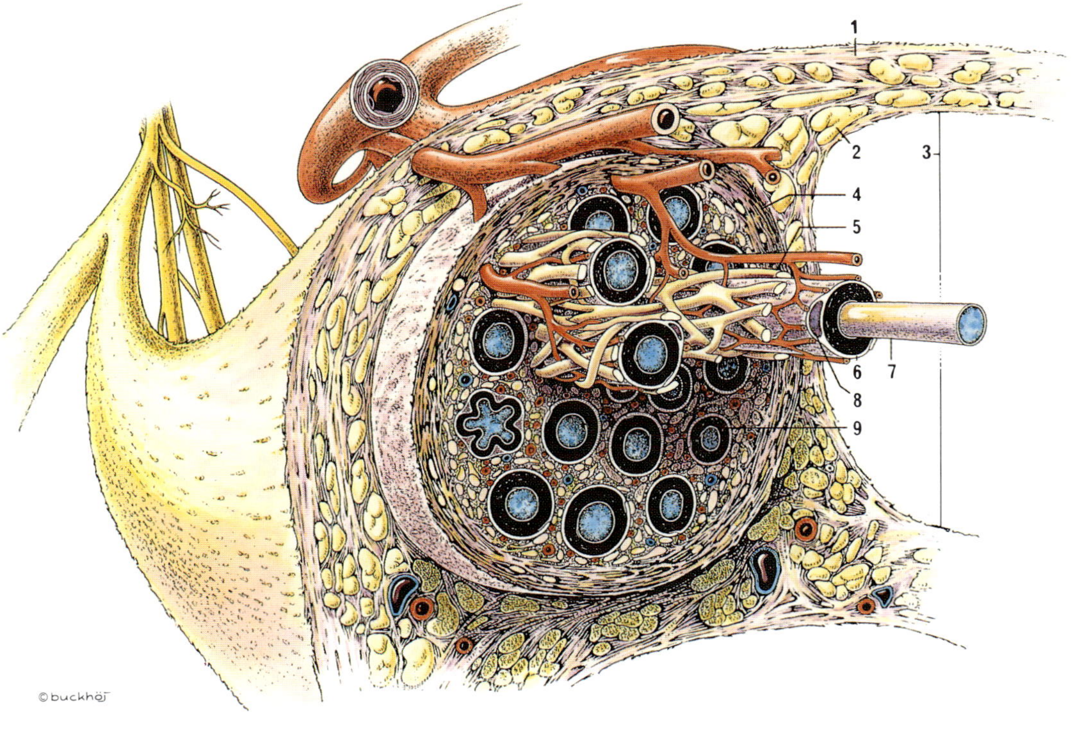

Because the spinal cord is shorter than the spine, the lower nerve roots become longer and more angulated caudally. The lower lumbar, the sacral and the coccygeal nerve rootlets form, together with the filum terminale, the cauda equina below the termination of the cord (Fig. 1.27).

It is in this region where spinal blocks are performed as the needle cannot damage the spinal cord, and the rootlets forming the cauda equina can move easily in the CSF.

Within the subarachnoid space the spinal nerves are divided into small rootlets and are covered with a layer of pia mater only. This is in contrast to the epidural space, where they are large mixed nerves with a substantial amount of connective tissue both inside and outside the nerve (Figs. 1.9 and 1.26). This explains the much smaller doses of local anaesthetic required for spinal anaesthesia compared to epidural blockade.

Fig. 1.27.

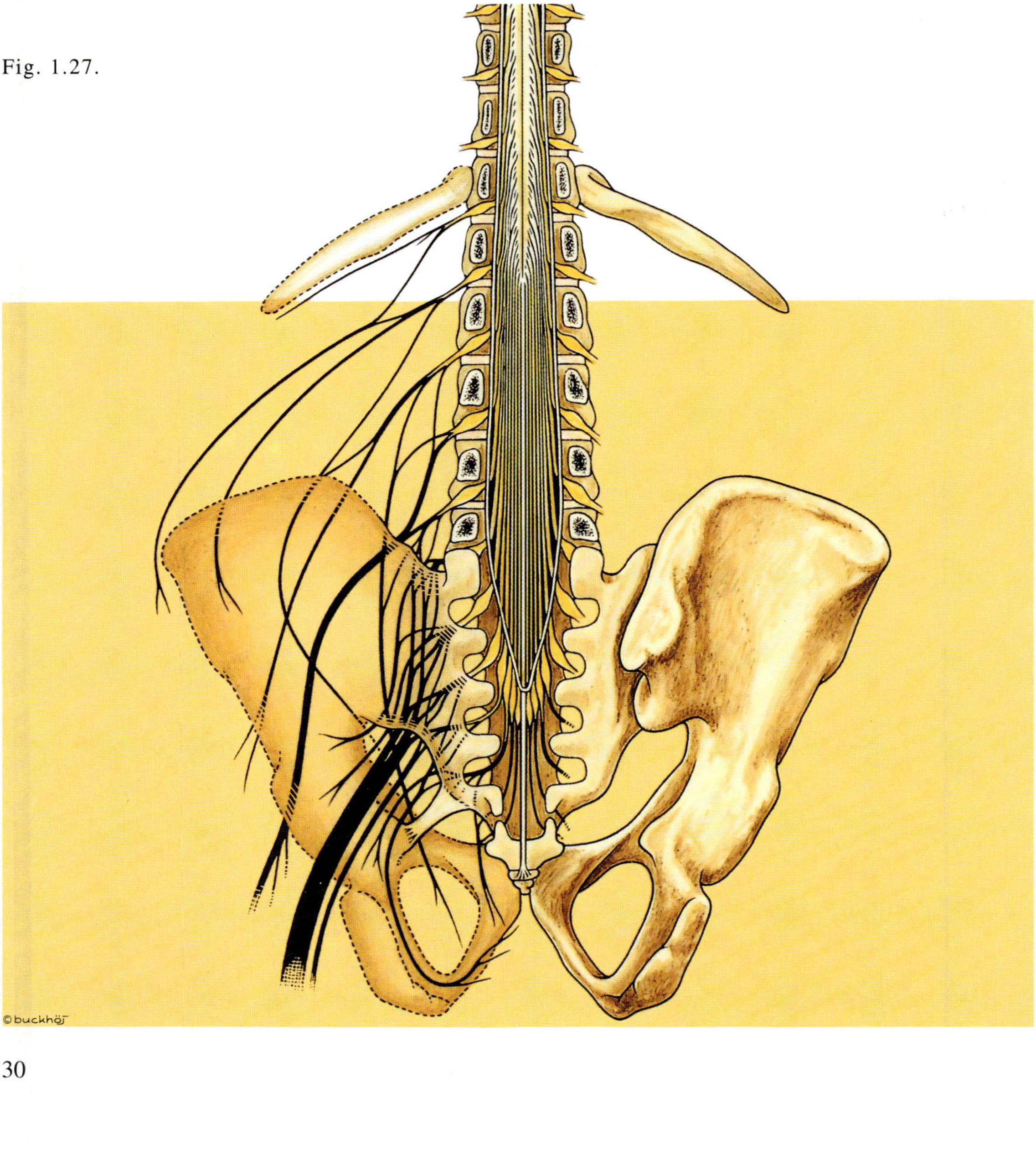

Segmental distribution of spinal nerves

The spinal nerves which leave the spinal canal through each intervertebral foramen quickly divide into anterior and posterior primary rami. The latter supply the skin and muscles of the back, and the former supply the rest of the body.

Each spinal segment supplies a specific region of the skin (dermatome), of muscle (myotome) and of bone (osteotome). In the cervical, brachial and lumbosacral regions, the anterior rami join to form nerve plexuses (Fig. 1.28).

In spinal anaesthesia, motor paralysis affects the movement of various joints and muscles. The segmental innervation of these is shown in the following list:

Shoulder	C6-8
Elbow	C5-8
Wrist	C6-7
Hand and digits	C7-8, T1
Intercostal	T1-11
Diaphragm	C3-5
Abdominal	T7-12
Hip, flexion	L1-3
Hip, extension	L5, S1
Knee, flexion	L5, S1
Knee, extension	L3-4
Ankle, flexion	L4-5
Ankle, extension	S1-2

The cutaneous distribution of the spinal nerves is shown in Fig. 1.29. It should be remembered that there is considerable overlap between adjacent spinal segments. The data were originally obtained from patients with spinal nerve injuries and depended upon clinical neurological observations and not anatomical dissection.

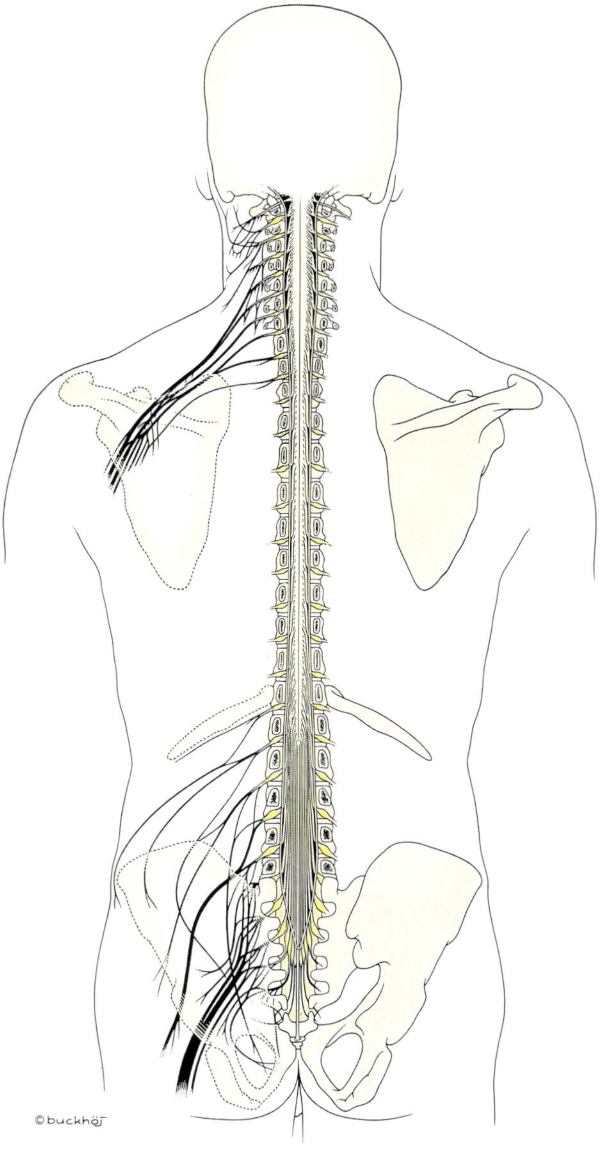

Fig. 1.28.

Fig. 1.29. Dermatomal distribution of spinal nerves. This fig is derived from several authorities and should be considered as a guide only.

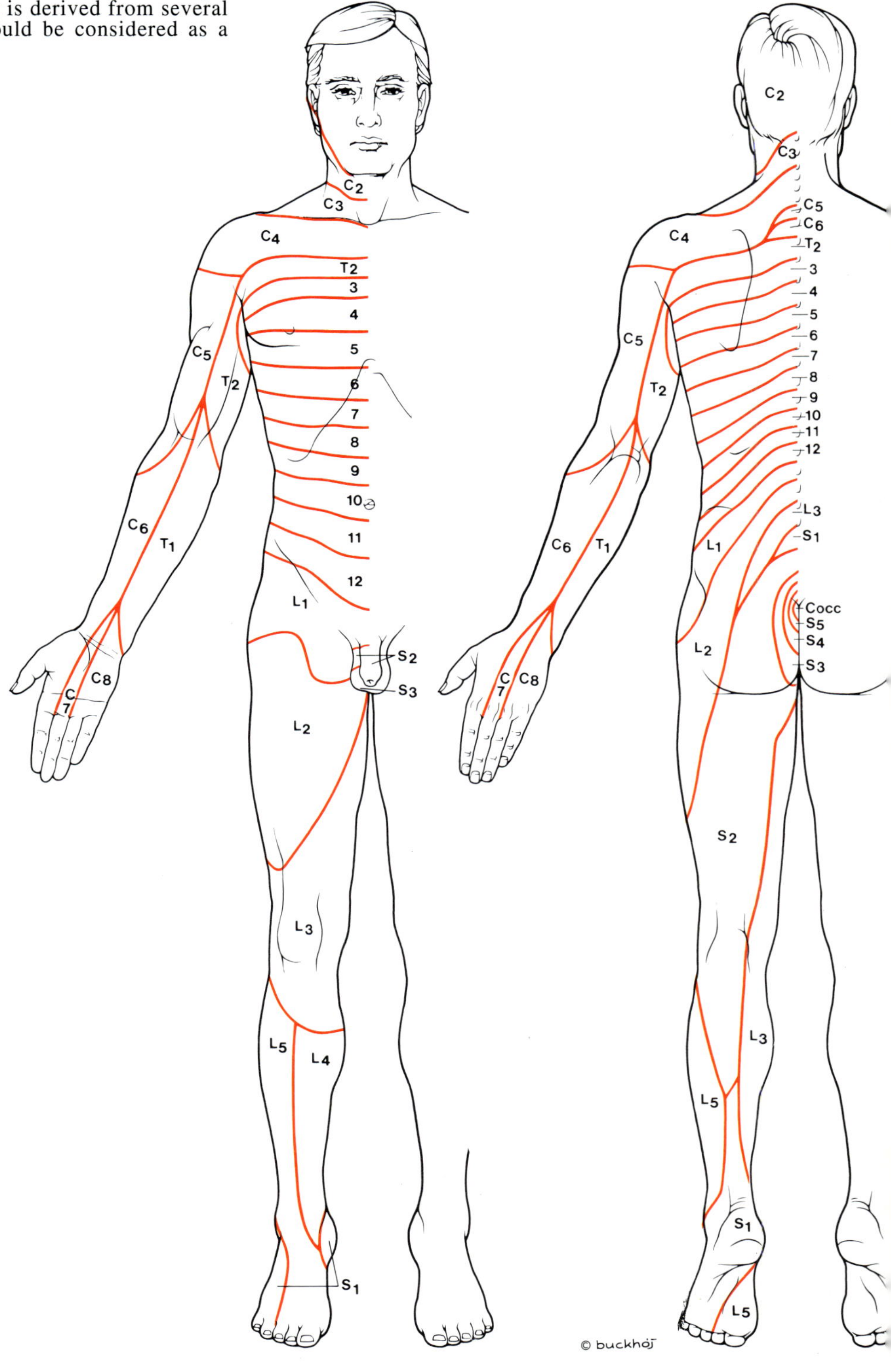

Autonomic nervous system

Spinal anaesthesia can cause a widespread blockade of both sympathetic and parasympathetic nerves. This has considerable effects, mainly on the control of the circulation but also on the normal function of the gastrointestinal tract (Fig. 1.30). In addition, afferent autonomic visceral nerves are involved in the appreciation of painful stimuli in the abdomen and must be blocked if total analgesia is to be achieved. Finally, blockade of the autonomic supply to endocrine glands can greatly modify the response of these glands to surgical stress (p. 128).

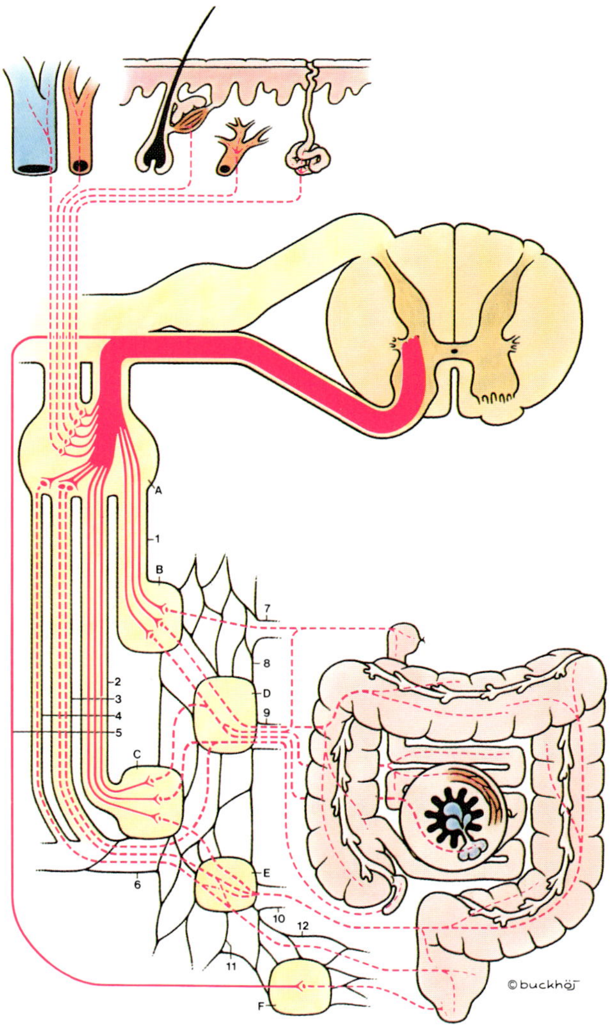

Fig. 1.30. Sympathetic efferent nerves.

A. Sympathetic ganglions from T6-L2
B. Coeliac ganglion
C. Superior mesenteric ganglion
D. Aorticorenal ganglion
E. Inferior mesenteric ganglion
F. Pelvic ganglion

1.	Greater splanchnic nerve	T6-9
2.	Lesser splanchnic nerve	T10-11
3.	Lowest splanchnic nerve	T12
4.	First lumbar splanchnic nerve	L1-2
5.	Pudendal nerve	S2-4
6.	Plexus surrounding gastroduodenal artery	
7.	Coeliac plexus	
8.	Superior mesenteric plexus	
9.	Superior hypogastric plexus	
10.	Inferior mesenteric plexus	
11.	Superior hypogastric plexus	
12.	Inferior hypogastric plexus (pelvic plexus)	

Sympathetic nervous system

Efferent impulses from the central nervous system to the blood vessels and organs supplied by sympathetic nerves must travel along both preganglionic and postganglionic nerves. Thus two nerve fibres are involved with a connecting synapse within a ganglion. The ganglia are located in the sympathetic chain, and in the large plexuses within the thorax and abdomen, such as the cardiac, coeliac and hypogastric plexuses.

Preganglionic nerve fibres arise from nerve cells in the lateral column of the grey matter of the spinal cord. They leave the spinal cord through the ventral nerve roots from T1 to L2. Some authorities claim that they may also arise in the cervical spinal nerves. Just lateral to the intervertebral foramina, the preganglionic nerve fibres, which are lightly myelinated, leave the spinal nerves to become the white rami communicantes which run to the sympathetic chain. Within the chain they may pass up or down to reach a synapse within the appropriate ganglion. Many do not synapse in the chain but leave it to reach ganglia in the large plexuses.

The sympathetic chain runs the length of the spinal column along the anterolateral aspect of the vertebral bodies (Figs. 1.22 and 1.31). In the cervical region the collections of ganglia make up the superior cervical, the middle cervical and the stellate ganglia. In the thorax the sympathetic chain gives rise to the splanchnic nerves (greater, lesser and lowest), which penetrate the diaphragm to reach the ganglia within the coeliac and aorticorenal plexuses. In the abdomen there are connections with the coeliac, aortic and hypogastric plexuses. The chain ends in the pelvis on the anterior surface of the sacrum. The unmyelinated postganglionic fibres arising from the ganglia are widely distributed to all the organs receiving a sympathetic nerve supply. Many run back to the spinal nerves via the grey rami communicantes and reach structures within the distribution of those spinal nerves, e.g. supply the blood vessels as well as organs within the skin, such as the sweat glands. Postganglionic nerves from the stellate ganglia are distributed to the head along the major blood vessels. While only 14 pairs of spinal nerves (T1-L2) give rise to preganglionic nerves, all spinal nerves receive postganglionic fibres.

The viscera receive their postganglionic fibres more directly through branches which leave the large plexuses. The segmental distribution of the visceral sympathetic nerves is shown in Table 1.1.

Table 1.1.

Head, neck and upper limbs	T1-5
Heart	T1-5
Lungs	T2-4
Oesophagus (lower end)	T5-6
Stomach	T6-10
Small intestine	T9-10
Large bowel	T11-L2
Liver and gallbladder	T7-9
Pancreas and spleen	T6-10
Kidney and ureter	T10-L2
Adrenal glands	T8-L1
Testis and ovary	T10-11
Bladder	T11-L2
Prostate	T11-L1
Uterus (uterine tube)	T10-L1

Fig. 1.31. Sympathetic efferent nerves.

1. Superior cervical ganglion
2. Middle cervical ganglion
3. Stellate ganglion
4. Coeliac ganglion
5. Superior mesenteric ganglion
6. Inferior mesenteric ganglion
7. Superior hypogastric plexus

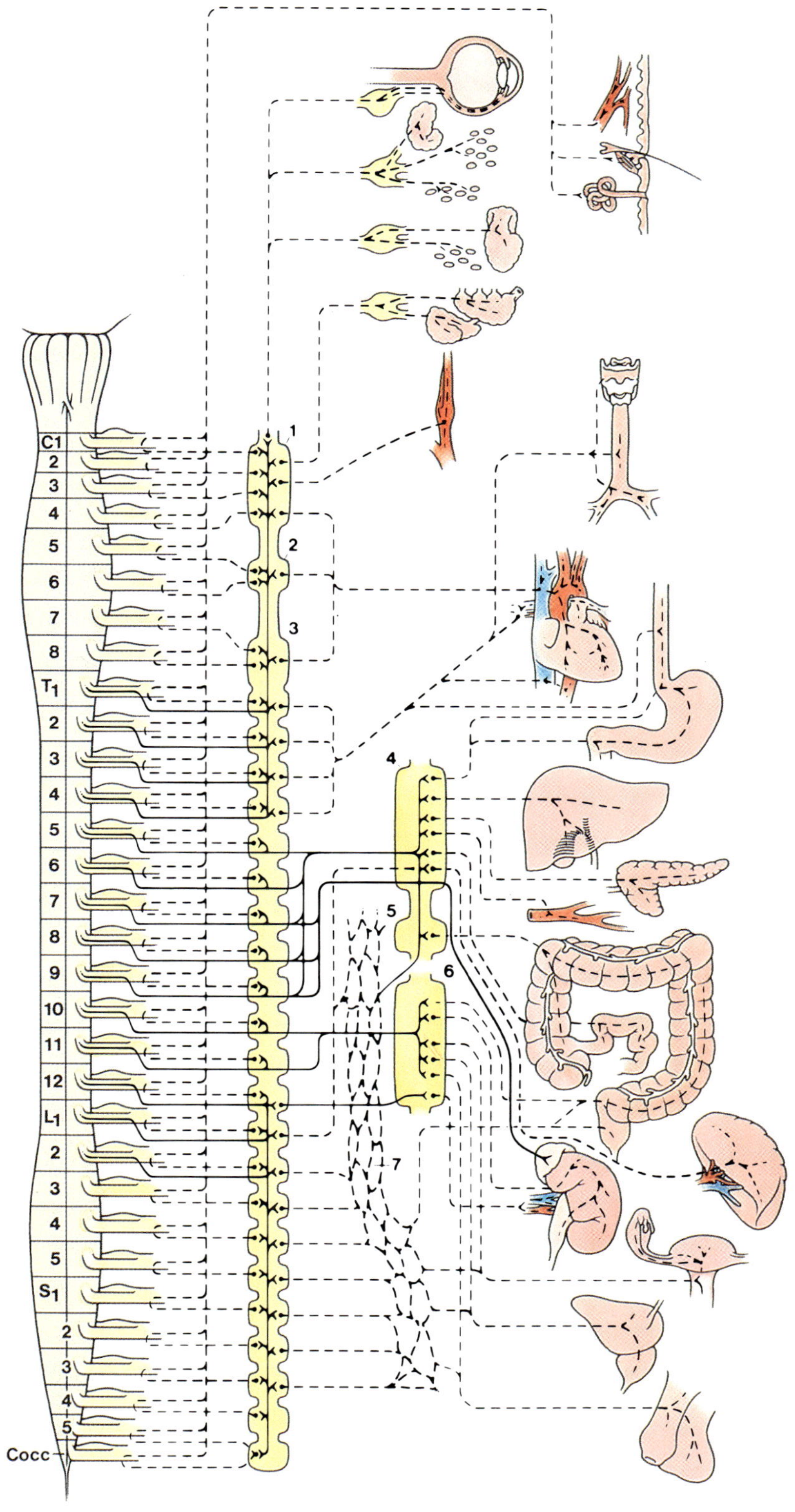
C1
2
3
4
5
6
7
8
T1
2
3
4
5
6
7
8
9
10
11
12
L1
2
3
4
5
S1
2
3
4
5
Cocc
1
2
3
4
5
6
7
©buckhöj

Parasympathetic nervous system

Efferent and afferent nerves of the parasympathetic system run either in cranial nerves (the cranial outflow) or in the 2nd, 3rd and 4th sacral nerves (the sacral outflow) (Fig. 1.32 and 33). The vagus nerve is the most important cranial nerve carrying parasympathetic efferent nerves, but these also exist in the oculomotor, the facial, the glossopharyngeal and the accessory nerves. Preganglionic fibres run all the way to the various organs they supply. Synapses occur in the walls of these organs with very short postganglionic fibres.

The vagus nerve supplies the heart, lungs, oesophagus and gastrointestinal tract down to the transverse colon. The sacral parasympathetic nerves are distributed with the corresponding sympathetic nerves to the large bowel below the transverse colon, the bladder, the sphincters and the reproductive organs.

Unlike all other autonomic nerves, the cranial parasympathetic nerves, and especially the vagus nerve, cannot be affected by spinal blockade unless local anaesthetic diffuses into the cranium.

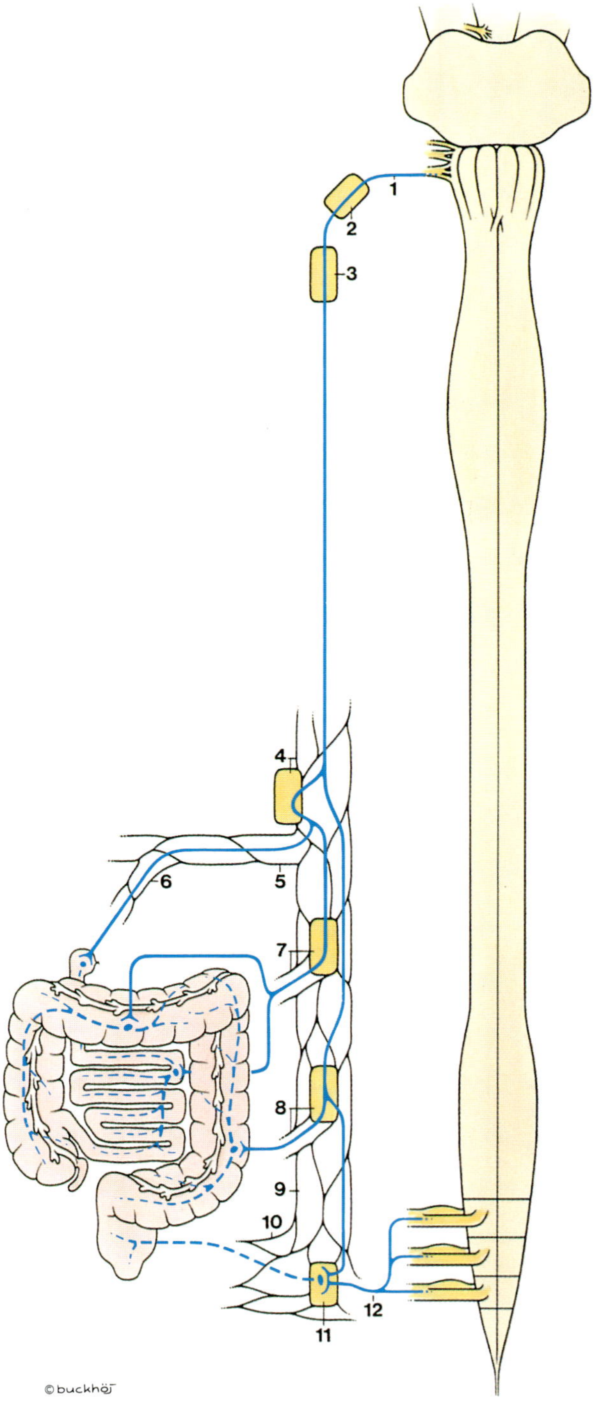

Fig. 1.32. Schematic diagram of the efferent component of the parasympathetic nervous system to the small and large intestines.

1. Vagus nerve
2. Superior vagal ganglion
3. Inferior vagal ganglion
4. Coelic ganglion and plexus
5. Hepatic plexus surrounding the common hepatic artery
6. Plexus surrounding gastroduodenal aretery
7. Superior mesenteric ganglion and plexus
8. Inferior mesenteric ganglion and plexus
9. Superior hypogastric plexus
10. Inferior hypogastric plexus (pelvic plexus)
11. Pelvic ganglion
12. Pelvic splanchnic nerves (nervi erigentes)

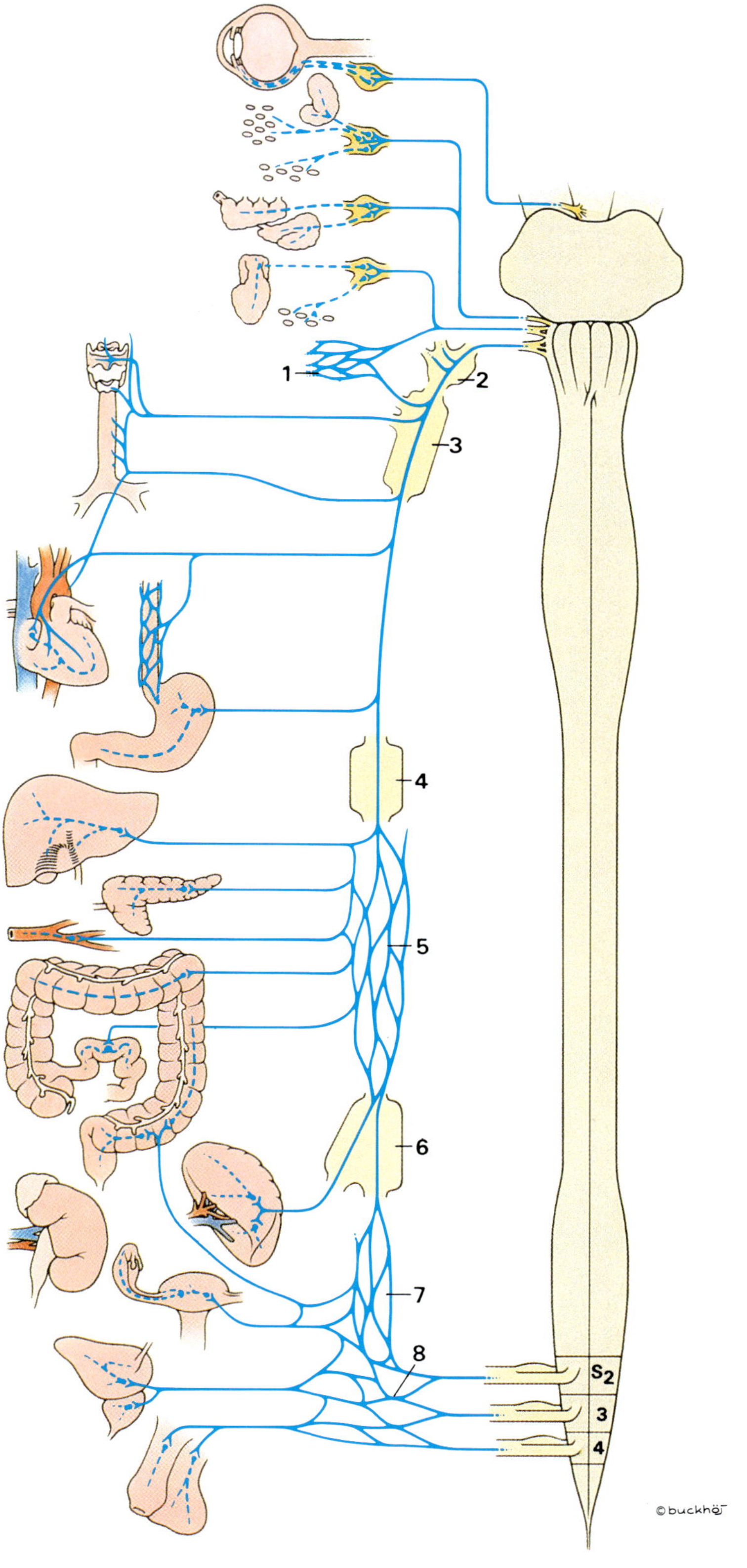

Fig. 1.33. Schematic diagram of the efferent components of the parasympathetic nervous system.

1. Pharyngeal plexus
2. Superior vagal ganglion
3. Inferior vagal ganglion
4. Coeliac ganglion
5. Coeliac plexus
6. Mesenteric ganglion
7. Superior hypogastric plexus
8. Inferior hypogastric plexus

Autonomic (visceral) afferent nerves

Distributed with the efferent nerves of both the sympathetic and parasympathetic systems are afferent fibres whose nerve cells are located in the dorsal root ganglia (Figs. 1.34 and 35). These fibres are responsible for the afferent arcs of visceral reflexes. They are concerned with sensations such as hunger, nausea, bladder distension and uterine contractions. Certain kinds of pain are mediated through these nerves, such as colic and labour pain. They are usually activated by excessive stretching or contraction of unstriated muscle but may also respond to inflammation (e.g. peritonitis) or ischaemia (e.g. angina).

Fig. 1.34. Schematic diagram of afferent sympathetic pathways from the heart.

1. Superior cervical ganglion
2. Middle cervical ganglion
3. Stellate ganglion

Fig. 1.35. Afferent parasympathetic nerve pathways from the stomach via the vagus nerve.

1. Superior vagal ganglion
2. Inferior vagal ganglion

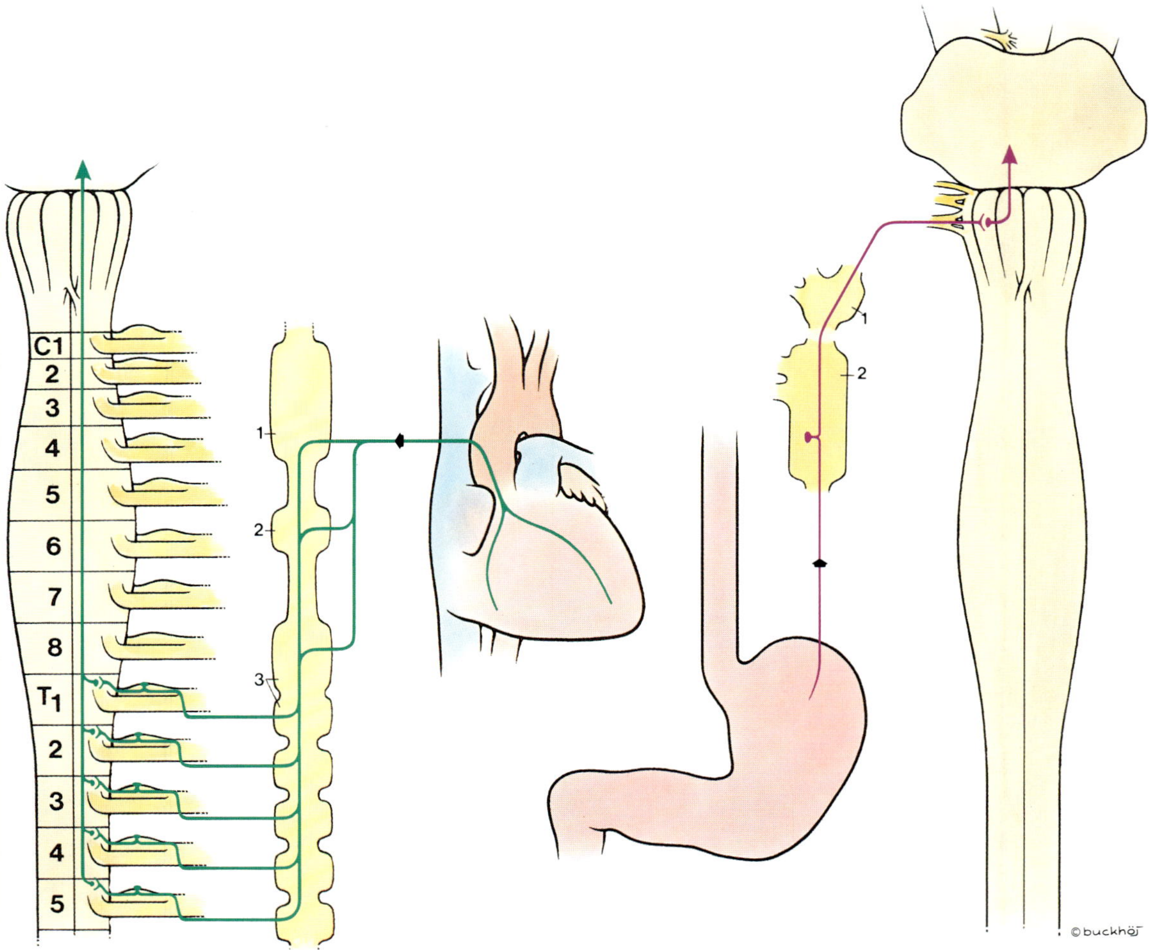

Cerebrospinal fluid

Both the brain and the spinal cord are enclosed in a fluid compartment, namely the subarachnoid space (Fig. 1.36). This serves as protection against trauma due to sudden movement. It also supports the brain and cord, and maintains a uniform pressure upon them. The effective weight of the brain is greatly reduced because it is immersed in fluid and the stress on its mechanical supports is evenly distributed.

Fig. 1.36. Cerebrospinal fluid circulation. Arrows indicate direction of flow of the cerebrospinal fluid.

1. Arachnoid granulation
2. Dura mater (outer layer)
3. Dura mater (inner layer)
4. Subdural space
5. Arachnoid mater
6. Subarachnoid space
7. Superior sagittal sinus
8. Pia mater
9. Choroid plexus of the 3rd ventricle
10. Great cerebral vein
11. Cisterna cerebellomedullaris
12. Interventricular foramen
13. Interpeduncular cistern
14. Aqueduct of Sylvius
15. Cistern of the great cerebral vein (cisterna ambiens)
16. Choroid plexus of the 4th ventricle
17. Foramen of Magendie

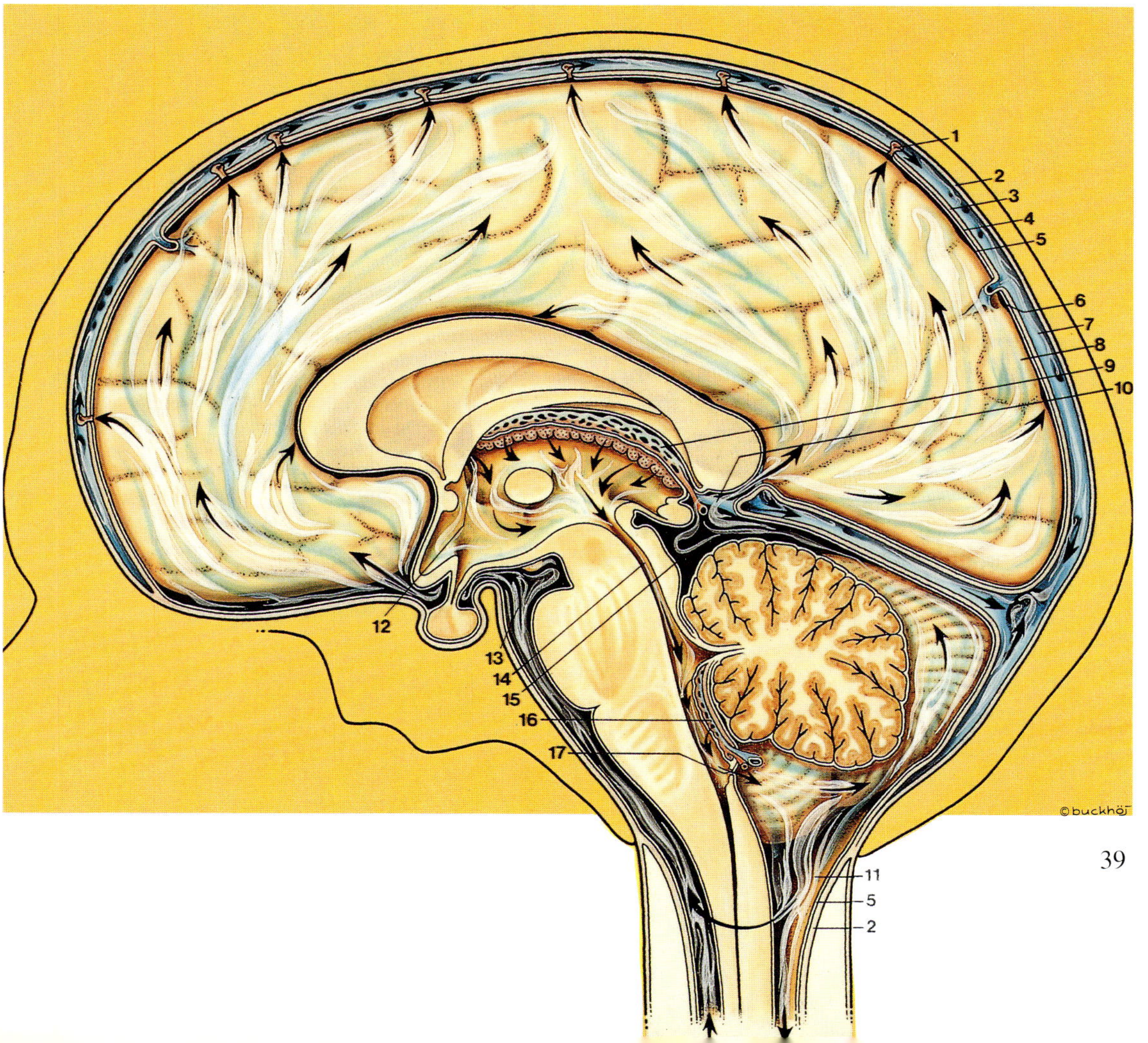

Microscopically the choroid plexus is made up of fringes which are collections of large numbers of villous processes, each with its own blood and nerve supply. Together the villous processes create a very large surface area from which CSF is secreted. The tela choroidea receives its blood supply from the choroidal branches of the internal carotid and the posterior cerebral arteries.

After passing into the cranial subarachnoid space, CSF rises over the surface of the brain through the gap in the tentorium cerebelli. The arachnoid granulations are small diverticula of the subarachnoid space which protrude into the sagittal and other venous sinuses (Fig. 1.39). As they grow with age they cause pitting of the skull due to resorption of bone. Arachnoid granulations are enlargements of arachnoid villi, which are present in large numbers in young subjects. Histologically the mesothelial cells of the arachnoid mater penetrate the dura and fuse with the endothelial lining of the venous sinuses. Each villus has a minute but direct connection with the lumen of the venous sinus, through a fine tubule.

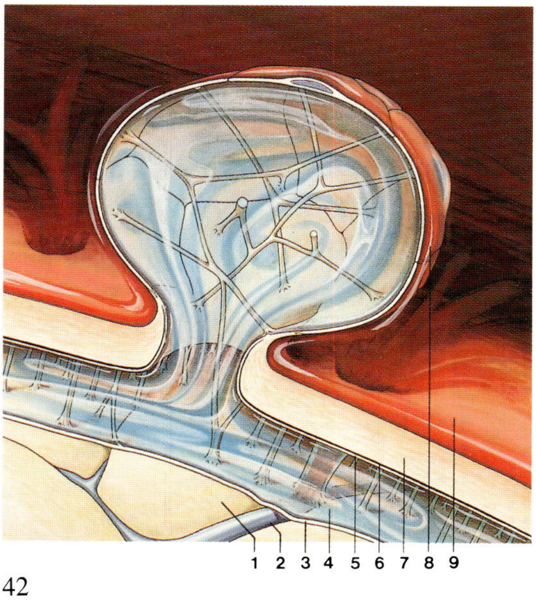

Fig. 1.39. Anatomy of an arachnoid granulation.

1. Cerebral cortex
2. Superficial cerebral vein
3. Pia mater
4. Subarachnoid space
5. Arachnoid mater
6. Subdural space
7. Dura mater (inner layer)
8. Arachnoid granulation
9. Superior sagittal sinus

References

The standard reference book used for this chapter was Gray´s Anatomy, 35th edition, eds. Warwick R and Williams PL, Longman, Edinburgh 1973.

1. Fink BR, Walker S. Orientation of fibers in human dorsal lumbar dura mater in relation to lumbar puncture. Anesth Analg 1989; 69:768

2. Reimann AF, Anson BI. Vertebral level of termination of the spinal cord, with a report of a case of sacral cord. Anat Rec 1944; 88:127

Chapter 2

Physiological considerations

Cerebrospinal fluid

Cerebrospinal fluid (CSF) is a clear colourless fluid whose physicochemical properties are shown in Table 2.1. Ninety percent of CSF is formed in the choroid plexus (small reddish tufts or patches of tissue) in the lateral, third and fourth ventricles (Fig. 1.38), while ten percent is derived from brain substance.[1] The blood and CSF are separated by impermeable "tight junctions" between epithelial cells (Fig. 2.1). The epithelial cells transfer certain molecules from the capillary side into the cerebral ventricles (Fig. 2.2). Water molecules in the epithelial cells dissociate into hydrogen and hydroxyl ions and the hydroxyl ions combine with carbon dioxide which is a product of cell metabolism. At the basolateral cell surface, hydrogen ions are exchanged for extracellular sodium ions from plasma. The sodium ions are actively pumped through the apical surface of the cell into the ventricles.

Table 2.1. Physicochemical properties of CSF.

Property	Value
Specific gravity	1.003-1.009
Density	1.0001-1.0005 (37°C)
Baricity*	1.000
pH***	7.31-7.34
Glucose***	50-75 mg·d L^{-1}
Protein***	18-41 mg·d L^{-1}
Total cell count***	2-5 μL^{-1}
Sodium***	137-153 mmol·L^{-1}
Potassium***	2.6-3.3 mmol·L^{-1}
Calcium***	1.02-1.34 mmol·L^{-1}
Magnesium***	0.9-1.2 mmol·L^{-1}
Chloride***	120-130 mmol·L^{-1}
Pressure**, ***	9-20 cm water

* For definition of baricity see Chapter 3
** Lateral recumbent position
*** From Geigy Scientific Tables (1981) Vol 1, 165-177.

Fig. 2.1. Essential nutrients reach the neurons and glial cells in the brain by crossing either the blood-CSF barrier, which is regulated by the choroid plexus, or the blood-brain barrier of the cerebral capillaries. Water-soluble molecules cannot diffuse freely between the blood and the CSF because of impermeable tight-junction seals between the choroid epithelial cells; instead the epithelial cells transfer certain molecules from one side of the barrier to the other. Once molecules enter the CSF, they diffuse through the "leaky" ependymal layer and reach the interstitial fluid around the neurons and glial cells.

Fig. 2.1a
1. Endothelial cell
2. Tight junction
3. Cerebral capillary
4. Neuron
5. Glucose
6. Interstitial fluid
7. Glial cell
8. Ependymal layer

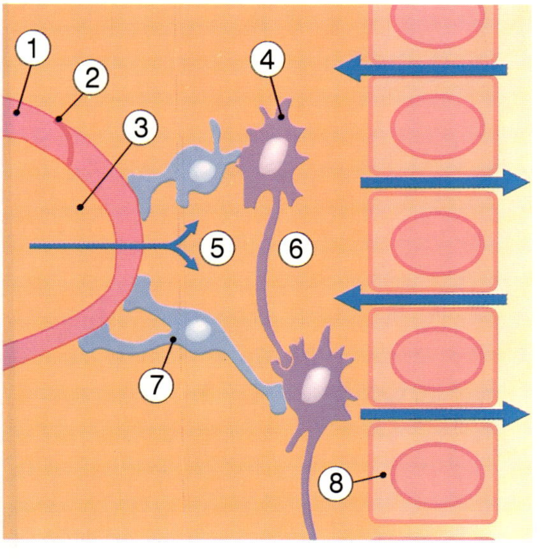

Fig. 2.1b
1. Choroid plexus, epithelial cell
2. Capillary
3. Tight junction
4. Ependymal layer

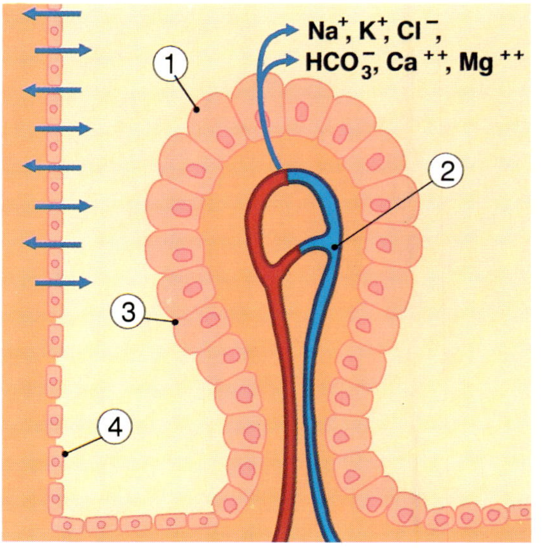

This is accompanied by a compensatory movement of chloride and bicarbonate ions into the CSF. To maintain osmotic equilibrium, water moves into the ventricles (Fig. 2.2).[1]

The volume of CSF formed daily is believed to be equal to the volume present in the central nervous system (CNS), which is approximately 150 mL. However, when CSF is lost (e.g. during and after lumbar puncture), considerable amounts can be produced to compensate for the loss.[2]

The rate of CSF absorption is pressure dependent and linear over a wide range. The arachnoid villi (granulations) situated in the cranial venous sinuses, drain the major portion of CSF.[3] When CSF pressure exceeds that in the venous sinus, fine tubules in the villi allow CSF to flow into the sinus. Conversely, when venous sinus pressure exceeds CSF pressure, the tips of the villi close, preventing reverse flow (Fig. 2.3).[1] Other possible sites of absorption include veins in the subarachnoid space and in lymphatic vessels of the cranial and spinal nerves.

Apart from the physical protection provided to the brain, CSF provides a chemically stable environment. The separation of blood and CSF compartmentalizes and regulates essential biochemical functions in the brain. In addition, it also probably takes part in nourishing the brain, and assists in removing the products of neuronal metabolism.[1] Likewise, it is important in the distribution and elimination of drugs injected into the CSF (e.g. local anaesthetics and opioids).

Fig. 2.2. Flow of ions across the blood-CSF barrier is regulated by several mechanisms in the choroid plexus.

1. Blood vessel (plasma)
2. Basolateral surface
3. Epithelial cell of choroid plexus
4. Tight junction
5. Ventricles
6. Apical surface
7. CSF in ventricle
8. Ion exchange

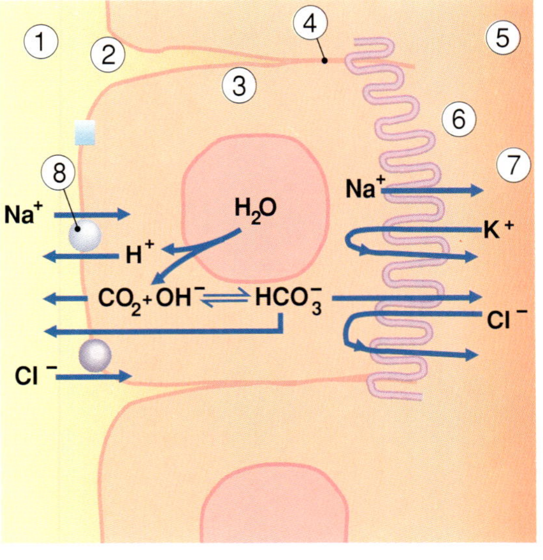

Fig. 2.3.

1. Superior sagital sinus
2. Endothelium
3. Falx cerebri
4. Arachnoid granulation
5. Superior cerebral vein
6. Cerebral cortex
7. Pia mater
8. Subarachnoid space and arachnoid trabecula
9. Arachnoid membrane
10. Subdural space
11. Meningeal vein
12. Venous lacuna
13. Dura mater
14. Diploic vein
15. Parietal bone (cranium)
16. Emissary vein
17. Pericraneum

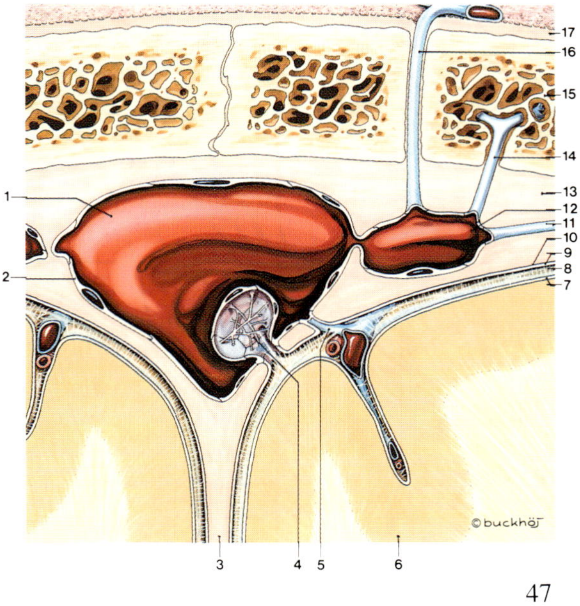

Spinomesencephalic tract (SMT)

SMT fibres (Fig. 2.8) terminate in the PAG and other mesencephalic nuclei. The SMT originates in laminae I and V and ascends both contralaterally and ipsilaterally (not shown). Some of the SMT neurons that terminate in the thalamus and limbic system are believed to have a discriminative, as well as autonomic, reflexive activity and motivational functions. In addition, the SMT, via its connections with the PAG, may activate descending inhibitory systems that produce analgesia.[17]

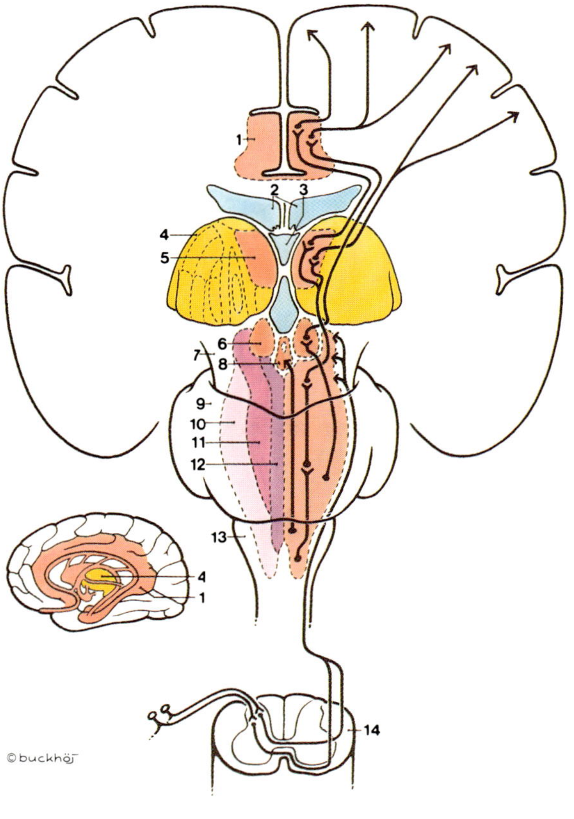

Fig. 2.8. Diagram showing the pathways followed by the spinomesencephalic tract from the spinal cord to the brain.

1. Limbic forebrain structure
2. Lateral ventricles
3. Third ventricle
4. Thalamus
5. Medial intralaminar thalamic nuclei
6. Hypothalamus
7. Mesencephalon
8. Periaqueductal grey (PAG)
9. Pons
10. Lateral reticular formation
11. Medial reticular formation
12. Median reticular formation
13. Medulla
14. Lumbar cord

Spinocervical tract (SCT)

The SCT is located in the dorsolateral funiculus and ascends ipsilaterally to terminate in the lateral cervical nucleus (Fig. 2.9). Fibres from the lateral cervical nucleus then cross to the contralateral thalamus. Similar to the neospinothalamic tract, the SCT is believed to be involved with spatial and temporal discrimination of pain stimuli.[18]

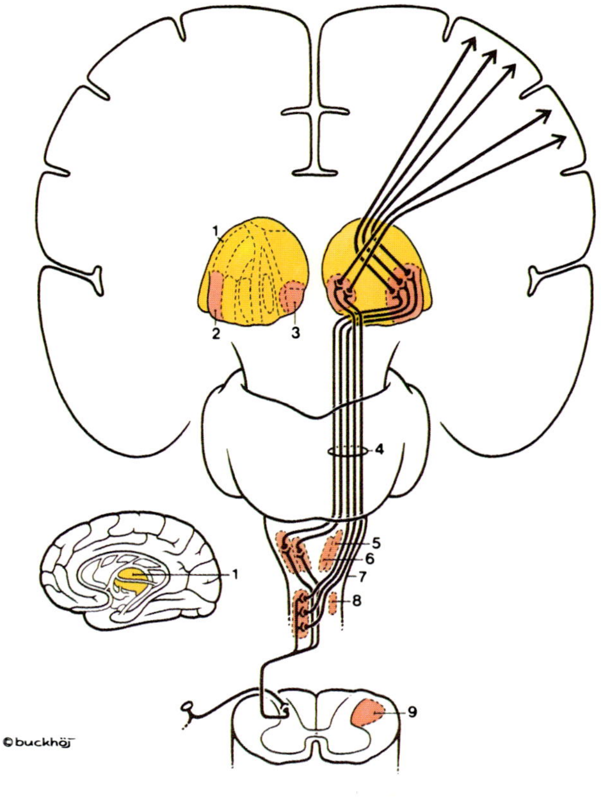

Fig. 2.9. Diagram showing the pathways followed by the spinocervical tract from the spinal cord to the brain.

1. Thalamus
2. Nucleus ventralis posterior lateralis
3. Posterior group of thalmic nuclei
4. Medial lemnicus
5. Nucleus cuneatus
6. Nucleus gracilis
7. Caudal medulla
8. Lateral cervical nucleus
9. Spinocervical tract

Descending pain control mechanisms

Stimulation of the PAG in the midbrain, either electrically or by microinjection of morphine, produces profound analgesia.[7-8] Projections from the PAG to the nucleus raphe magnus and to the medullary reticular formation nuclei descend via the dorsal lateral funiculus to the dorsal horn neurons (Fig. 2.4). These descending fibres are believed to release 5HT which suppresses the activation of SG cells(Fig. 2.5). In addition, descending fibres that originate in the locus coeruleus release norepinephrine, which also suppresses activation of cells in the SG.[9] The antinociceptive action of adrenergic agents is believed to be responsible for the analgesic effect of intraspinal clonidine.

Fig. 2.10. Structures involved in descending pain control mechanisms.

1. Right lateral ventricle
2. Third ventricle
3. Periaqueductal grey area
4. Locus coeruleus
5. Reticular formation
6. Nucleus raphe magnus
7. Fourth ventricle

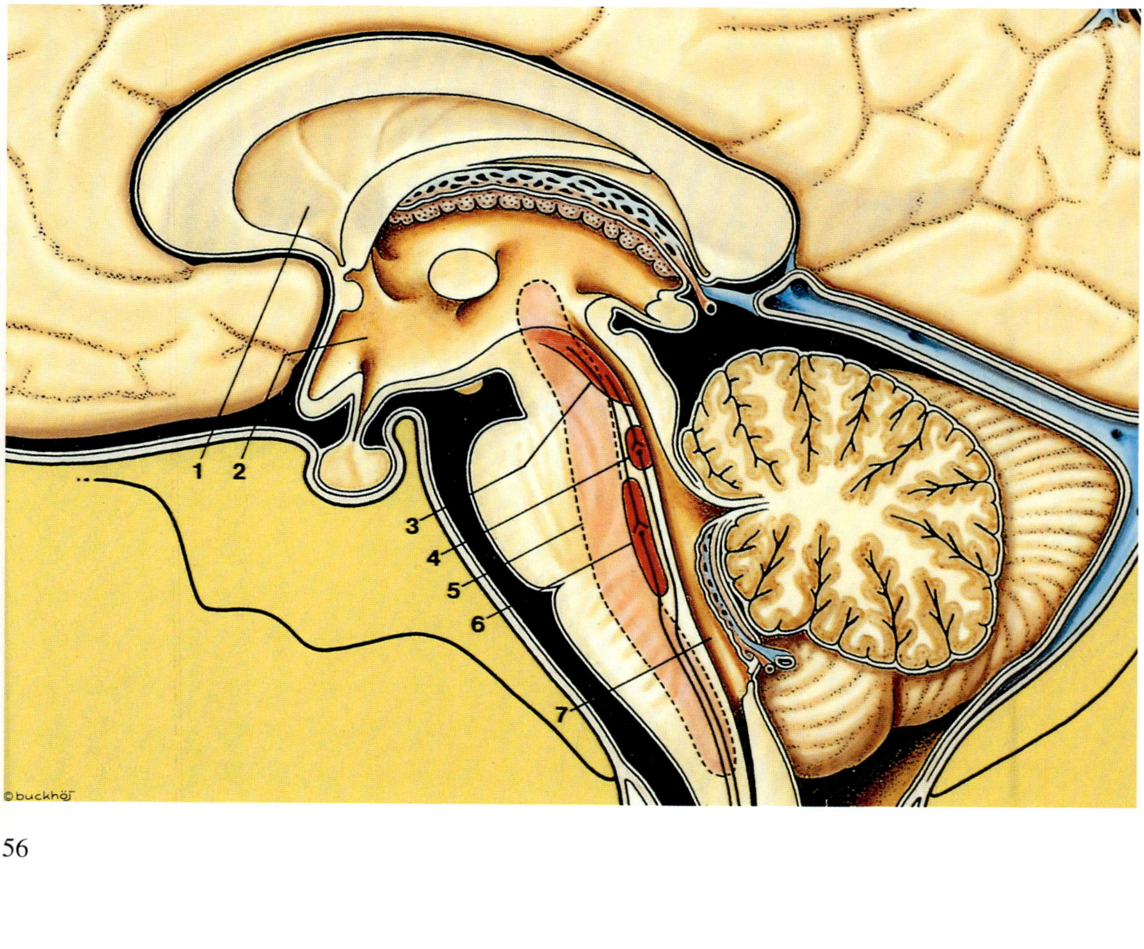

Visceral pain pathways

Autonomic afferent neurons from visceral organs to the brainstem and spinal cord are the visceral afferent components of the spinal and the cranial nerves. The cell bodies of these neurons, like those of the somatic afferent neurons, are located in the dorsal root ganglia of the respective nerves (Fig. 2.11). The visceral afferent nerve fibres traverse the autonomic ganglia but make no synaptic contacts in them and enter the spinal cord or the brainstem in association with the somatic afferent fibres of the same nerves. Both visceral and somatic afferent nerve fibres make reflex connections with the preganglionic autonomic neurons in the brainstem and spinal cord. They are, therefore, functionally related to the autonomic nerves but are not anatomical components of them.[19]
Visceral afferents converge on the dorsal horn neurons, as do somatic nociceptive afferents. Noxious visceral stimuli are conveyed together with noxious somatic stimuli by means of the spinothalamic pathways to the brain. Visceral pain is believed to result from high-frequency firing of visceral afferents which ordinarily mediate homeostatic rather than nociceptive functions. Thus, visceral afferents may fire at low rates in response to mild dilatation of a hollow viscus but fire at very high rates when excessive distension occurs. These high rates of discharge activate pain projection systems originating in the dorsal horn. The resulting pain is therefore perceived to originate from somatic regions whose neurones project to the same spinal cord segments.[20]

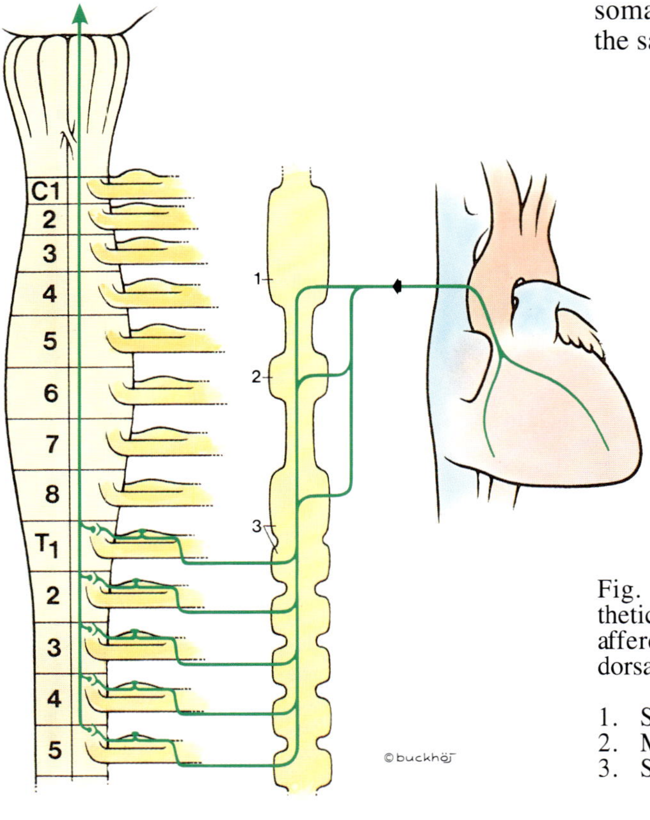

Fig. 2.11. Schematic diagram of afferent sympathetic pathways from the heart. Note that like all afferent nerves, the cell bodies lie within the dorsal root ganglia.

1. Superior cervical ganglion
2. Middle cervical ganglion
3. Stellate ganglion

Table 2.3 lists the viscera and their segmental nociceptive nerve supply. It is necessary to have an appreciation of the innervation of visceral structures when deciding on the level of spinal anaesthesia that will be adequate for surgery on these structures. For example, although the cutaneous innervation of the scrotum is of sacral origin, surgery upon the testes will require a spinal anaesthetic level extending at least to the T10 dermatome. This is because the visceral afferents associated with the testes travel with the sympathetic fibres entering the central nervous system at the T10 level. As another example, consider Caesarean section, which is said to require mid-thoracic levels of spinal anaesthesia to insure comfort for the patient. This is likely to be due to the fact that the visceral and parietal peritoneum is a large continuous structure. Traction on the uterus, for example, results in peritoneal irritation and pain when the spinal level does not extend high enough to block the peritoneal pain fibres entering the spinal cord at the most cephalad point. Sometimes, during abdominal operations and despite a high level of analgesia, the block is inadequate as patients experience ill-defined discomfort, nausea and vomiting. The cause is failure to block all fibres that carry sensation centrally, including the vagus nerve.

Table 2.3. Segmental distribution of sympathetic nerves.

Head, neck and upper limbs	T1-5
Heart	T1-5
Lungs	T2-4
Oesophagus	T5-6
Stomach	T6-10
Small intestine	T9-10
Large bowel	T11-L2
Liver and gallbladder	T7-9
Pancreas and spleen	T6-10
Kidney and ureter	T10-L2
Adrenal glands	T8-L1
Testis and ovary	T10-11
Bladder	T11-L2
Prostate	T11-L1
Uterus	T10-L1

Cardiovascular effects of spinal anaesthesia

Arterial hypotension of varying degrees is a common physiological manifestation of a successful spinal block. In one study of more than 11,000 cases, hypotension occurred in 38% of the patients.[21] The primary cause of arterial hypotension during spinal anaesthesia is the blockade of preganglionic sympathetic nerve fibres (Fig. 1.31). The degree of hypotension relates to the spread of the local anaesthetic agent within the subarachnoid space and the extent of the sympathetic blockade (Fig. 2.12).[22] For example a low block limited to the lumbar and sacral dermatomes causes little or no change in blood pressure. Spinal anaesthesia extending to the mid-thoracic level results in a moderate fall in blood pressure. High spinal anaesthesia results in sympathetic blockade of fibres innervating the heart as well as those controlling peripheral vascular beds and may thus produce profound hypotension. Sympathetic blockade usually extends to spinal segments above the sensory blockade. While it is generally held that the difference is 2 spinal segments[23-24]. recent studies show great variabillity in this regard. Some find as much as 6 segments´ difference,[25] while others show none.[26]

Fig. 2.12. Cardiovascular changes during spinal anaesthesia at different segmental levels. All patients are assumed to be horizontal. PR= peripheral resistance; HR=heart rate; CO=cardiac output; VR = central venous return; C=contractility; MAP=mean arterial pressure; NC=no change.

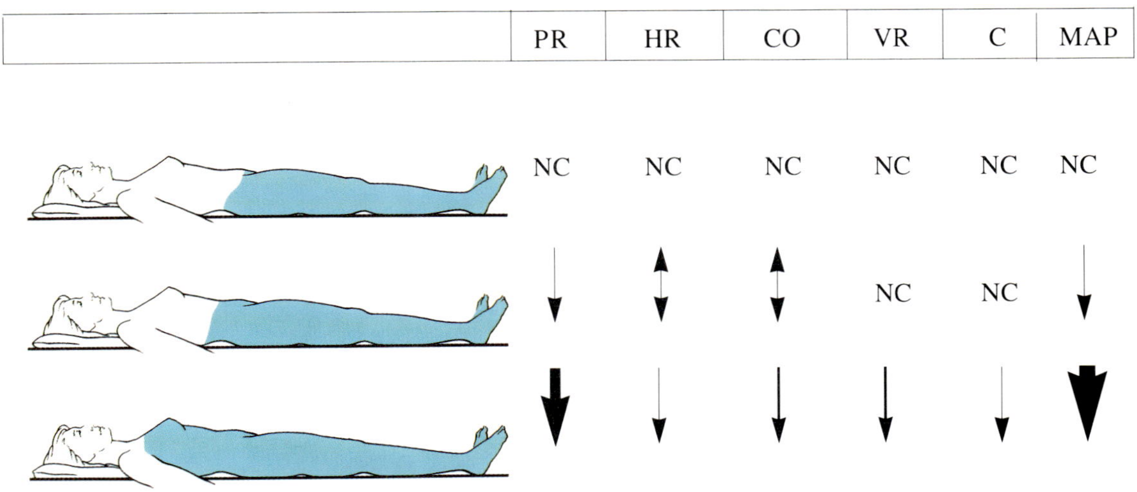

Physiological regulation of blood pressure

Blood pressure is determined by peripheral vascular resistance and cardiac output (Fig. 2.13). Cardiac output is a function of heart rate and stroke volume. Stroke volume is determined by the intrinsic contractility of cardiac muscle, the resistance against which the heart must contract (afterload) and the filling pressure within the left ventricle (preload), which is related to the venous return. Thus, changes in blood pressure relate directly to changes in either vascular resistance, cardiac output or both.[22] Cardiac output is affected by changes in preload, afterload, contractility and heart rate. Peripheral vascular resistance is controlled by the sympathetic innervation of the arterioles and by the local metabolic environment (tissue and blood pH, CO_2 and O_2 concentration). Thus, hypotension during spinal anaesthesia is related to the extent of sympathetic blockade, which influences peripheral vascular resistance and cardiac output.[27] The magnitude of the cardiovascular changes therefore depends upon the degree of sympathetic tone present immediately before the spinal injection.[28]

Fig. 2.13. The determinants of cardiac performance and arterial blood pressure.

Reproduced with permission from Mark and Steele.[22]

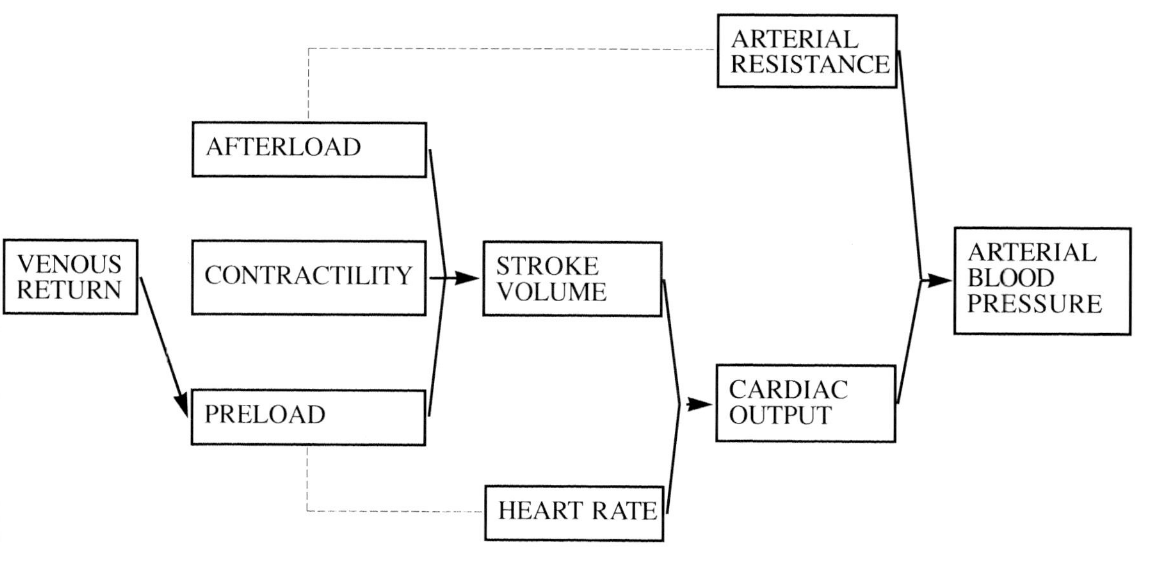

Peripheral vascular resistance

Sympathetic blockade limited to the lower thoracic or mid-thoracic region results in vasodilatation of the lower limbs with compensatory vasoconstriction in the upper limbs. Thus, peripheral vascular resistance only slightly decreases, limiting the degree of hypotension. As the block extends higher the vasodilatation increases while the ability to compensate by vasoconstriction decreases.[22]

Cardiac output

Spinal anaesthesia, which extends only to the mid-thoracic level, does not cause significant changes in cardiac output provided the patient remains horizontal or head down (Fig. 2.12). However, spinal anaesthesia which extends to the upper thoracic or cervical level may cause a significant reduction in cardiac output due to changes in heart rate, venous return and contractility.[22]

Heart rate

Sympathetic fibres from T1-T5 control cardiac rate. Spinal anaesthesia that blocks these fibres causes significant cardiac sympathetic denervation (Fig. 2.12). As there is normally a degree of sympathetic tone to the heart, this denervation causes a moderate decrease in heart rate.[29] The profound bradycardia observed in some patients during high spinal anaesthesia is probably due to enhanced vagal activity such as occurs during vasovagal syncope, or by intracardiac reflexes (vide infra).[30]

Stroke volume

Stroke volume may be reduced during high spinal anaesthesia by a reduction in venous return[22] and a decrease in cardiac contractility (Fig. 2.12).

Venous return

Venous return in sympathectomized patients is very dependent on gravity and therefore on posture (vide infra).[28]

The sympathetic control of the venous system is essential in maintaining venous return and therefore cardiovascular homeostasis during postural changes. The veins form a low pressure system and contain by far the largest proportion of the circulating blood (approximately 70%). When spinal anaesthesia produces sympathetic blockade, this control is lost and the venous return becomes gravity dependent.[31] If the lower limbs are below the right atrium, the denervated veins will dilate, sequestering a large volume of blood. The resultant decrease in venous return and thus cardiac output, together with the reduced peripheral resistance, can cause profound hypotension.

Contractility

Blockade of the sympathetic innervation of the heart can cause a decrease in inotropism leading to a modest (around 15%) reduction in cardiac output.

Syncope

Clinicians experienced with spinal anaesthesia recognize the clinical picture of rapidly developing hypotension and profound bradycardia, usually accompanied by nausea and sometimes vomiting. Momentary cardiac arrest and unconsciousness[32] can occur and sweating and pallor are common during recovery. It occurs only in conscious patients, and never in patients given concomitant general anaesthesia.[33] The resemblance to a vasovagal fainting attack is striking, and the vagus nerve may play a role.

The essential feature of syncope is a sudden failure of venous return leading to greatly reduced cardiac output.[34-36] The normal response to this is tachycardia and vasoconstriction to prevent venous dilatation. During syncope, bradycardia occurs, causing a rapid reduction in cardiac output. Fortunately sympathetic activity returns and provided there is no impediment to the venous return (e.g. by the head-up position or IVC occlusion), arterial pressure and heart rate increase. If unconsciousness occurs, recovery

Anaesthetic-related factors

The degree of hypotension may depend on the spinal anaesthetic agent. Despite achieving the same level of sensory anaesthesia, bupivacaine produced less hypotension than tetracaine.[42] The difference in hypotension may relate to greater sympathetic B-fibre blockade with tetracaine (as demonstrated in *in vitro* studies) compared to bupivacaine.[43]

The baricity of the anaesthetic solution may also affect hypotension during spinal anaesthesia. Hyperbaric solutions of tetracaine and bupivacaine result in more hypotension than isobaric or hypobaric solutions.[44,45] These differences probably relate to differences in the level of sensory and sympathetic block. Hyperbaric solutions spread further than isobaric or hypobaric solutions and cause more sympathetic blockade.

Concomitant general anaesthesia presumably increases the incidence of hypotension during spinal anaesthesia as this is known to occur when general anaesthesia is combined with epidural block (see p. 135).[46]

In summary, cardiovascular alterations are normal physiological responses during spinal anaesthesia and are due to sympathetic fibre blockade. Knowledge of the factors responsible for blood pressure changes makes it possible to avoid severe hypotension. Such knowledge is also valuable for choosing the appropriate treatment for cardiovascular depression, should it occur.

Respiratory effects of spinal anaesthesia

The effects of spinal anaesthesia on respiratory function relate to the level of conduction blockade. Spinal anaesthesia extending to the mid-thoracic level or lower, rarely causes significant alteration in pulmonary function. However, spinal anaesthesia that extends to the upper-thoracic dermatomes can cause detrimental changes in respiratory function (e.g. in patients with chronic obstructive airways disease).[47] On the other hand obese individuals may experience improved oxygenation, presumably due to increased chest wall compliance secondary to abdominal muscle paralysis.[48] Mid-thoracic spinal anaesthesia has no significant effect on tidal volume, respiratory rate, minute ventilation or end-tidal PCO_2. However, respiratory arrest can occur following accidental total spinal anaesthesia, due to paralysis of the respiratory muscles and/or brainstem ischaemia secondary to severe hypotension.[49]

Control of breathing

Studies in un-premedicated patients during spinal anaesthesia with isobaric bupivacaine and hyperbaric tetracaine show a decrease in resting end-tidal PCO_2 of approximately 0.3-0.7 kPa. CO_2 rebreathing increased minute ventilation and mouth occlusion pressure. The response to CO_2 during spinal anaesthesia is inversely correlated with age, i.e. younger patients have greater increases in minute ventilation than older patients.[50,51]

Spinal anaesthesia extending to mid to upper thoracic levels occasionally produces dyspnoea that is not caused by respiratory muscle weakness. The dyspnoea may originate in respiratory centres in the brain that are deprived of afferent input from the abdomen and chest wall during spinal anaesthesia. The drive to breathe is normally inhibited by these proprioceptive impulses. When they are blocked by high spinal anaesthesia there is an increased drive to breathe, causing a decrease in resting end-tidal PCO_2 and an increase in ventilatory responsiveness to CO_2. The patient may perceive this increased ventilatory drive as dyspnoea.[50,51]

References

1. Spector R, Johanson CE (1989) The mammalian choroid plexus. Sci Am 261: 68

2. Merritt HH, Fremont-Smith F (1938) The Cerebrospinal Fluid. Philadelphia: WB Saunders Co

3. McComb JG (1983) Recent research into the nature of cerebrospinal fluid formation and absorption. J Neurosurg 59: 369

4. Dubner R, Bennett GJ (1983) Spinal and trigeminal mechanisms of nociception. Annu Rev Neurosci 6: 381

5. Bonica JJ (1990) Anatomic and physiologic basis of nociception and pain. In: Bonica JJ, The Management of Pain, vol II. Philadelphia: Lea & Febiger p. 28

6. Rexed, B (1954) A cytoarchitectonic atlas of the spinal cord in the cat. J Comp Neurol 100: 297

7. Reynolds DV (1969) Surgery in the rat during electrical analgesia induced by focal brain stimulation. Science 164: 444

8. Mayer DJ, Wolfle TL, Akil H, Carder B, Liebesking JC (1971) Analgesia from electrical stimulation in the brainstem of the rat. Science 174:1351

9. Westlund KN, Coulter JD (1980) Descending projections of the locus coeruleus and subcoeruleus/medial parabrachial nuclei in monkey: axonal transport studies and dopamine-beta-hydroxylase immunocytochemistry. Brain Res 2: 235

10. Lamotte C, Pert CB, Snyder SH (1976) Opiate receptor binding in primate spinal cord: distribution and changes after dorsal root section. Brain Res 112: 407

11. Yaksh TL, Hammond DL (1982) Peripheral and central substrates involved in the rostrad transmission of nociceptive information. Pain 13: 1

12. Ruda MA, Bennett GJ, Dubner R. (1986) Neurochemistry and neural circuitry in the dorsal horn. Prog Brain Res 66: 219

13. Willis WD, Coggeshall RE (1978) Sensory mechanisms of the spinal cord. NY, Plenum

14. Melzack R, Wall PD (1965) Pain mechanisms: a new theory. Science 150: 971

15. Willis WD, Kenshalo DR Jr, Leonard RD (1979) The cells of origin of the primate spinothalamic tract. J Comp Neurol 188: 543

16. Kevetter GA, Haber LH, Yesierski RP, Chung JM, Martin RF, Willis WD (1982) Cells of origin of the spinoreticular tract in the monkey. J Comp Neurol 207: 61

17. Hylden JL, Hayashi H, Bennett GJ (1986) Lamina I spinomesencephalic neurons in the cat ascend via the dorsolateral funiculi. Somatosens Res 4: 31

18. Truex RC, Taylor MJ, Smyth MQ, Gildenberg PL (1970) The lateral cervical nucleus of cat, dog and man. J Comp Neurol 139: 93

19. Netter FH (1962) The Nervous System. NJ: CIBA p. 82

20. Cousins, MJ. Visceral pain. In: Anderson S, Bond M, Mehta M, Swerdlow M, eds (1987) Chronic Non Cancer Pain: Assessment and Practical Management. Lancaster: MTP Press

21. Moore DC (1966) Spinal subarachnoid block. JAMA 195: 123

22. Mark JB, Steele SM (1989) Cardiovascular effects of spinal anesthesia. Int Anesthesiol Clin 27: 31

23. Greene NM (1958) The area of differential block during spinal anesthesia with hyperbaric tetracaine. Anesthesiology 19: 45

24. Brull SJ, Greene NM (1989) Time-courses of zones of differential sensory blockade during spinal anesthesia with hyperbaric tetracaine or bupivacaine. Anesth Analg 69: 342

25. Chamberlain DP, Chamberlain BD (1986) Changes in the skin temperature of the trunk and their relationship to sympathetic blockade during spinal anesthesia. Anesthesiology 65: 139

26. Malmqvist LA, Bengtsson M, Björnsson G, Jorfeldt L, Löfsftröm JB (1987) Sympathetic activity and haemodynamic variables during spinal analgesia in man. Acta Anaesthesiol Scand 31: 467

27. Greene NM (1981) Preganglionic sympathetic blockade in man: a study of spinal anesthesia. The Torsten Gordh Lecture, 1980. Acta Anaesthesiol Scand 25: 463

28. Pugh LGC, Wyndham CL (1950) The circulatory effects of high spinal anesthesia in hypertensive and control subjects. Clin Sci 9: 189

29. Greene NM (1981) Physiology of Spinal Anesthesia, 3rd ed. Baltimore: Williams & Wilkins p. 93

30. Greene NM (1981) Physiology of Spinal Anesthesia, 3rd ed. Baltimore: Williams & Wilkins p. 98

31. Greene NM (1981) Physiology of Spinal Anesthesia, 3rd ed. Baltimore: Williams & Wilkins p. 121

32. Mackey DC, Carpenter RL, Thompson GE, Brown DL, Bodily MN (1989) Bradycardia and asystole during spinal anesthesia: a report of three cases without morbidity. Anesthesiology 70:866

33. Scott DB (1982) Cardiovascular effects of lumbar epidural and spinal anesthesia. Reg Anesth (Suppl) 7:S21

34. Öberg B, Thorén P (1972) Increased activity in left ventricular receptors during hemorrhage or occlusion of caval veins in the cat. A possible cause of the vaso-vagal reaction. Acta Physiol Scand 85:164

35. Sanders JS, Ferguson DW (1989) Profound sympathoinhibition complicating hypovolemia in humans. Ann Int Med 111:439

36. Weissler AM, Warren JV, Estes EH, McIntosh HD, Leonard JJ (1957) Vassodepressor syncope. Factors indluencing cardiac output. Circulation 15:875

37. Abboud FM (1989) Ventricular syncope. Is the heart a sensory organ? NEJM 320:390

38. Ward RJ, Kennedy W, Bonica JJ, Martin WE, Tolas AG, Akamatsu T (1966) Experimental evaluation of atropine and vasopressors for the treatment of hypotension of high subarachnoid anesthesia. Anesth Analg 45:621

39. Lewis T (1931) Vasovagal syncope and the carotid sinus mechanism. Br Med J 1:873

40. Wildsmith JA (1989) Predicting the spread of spinal anaesthesia. Br J Anaesth 62: 353

41. Defalque RJ (1962) Compared effects of spinal and extradural anesthesia upon the blood pressure. Anesthesiology 23: 627

42. Bigler D, Hjortsø NC, Edström H, Christensen NJ, Kehlet H (1986) Comparative effects of intrathecal bupivacaine and tetracaine on analgesia, cardiovascular function and plasma catecholamines. Acta Anaesthesiol Scand 30: 199

43. Gissen AJ, Covino BG, Gregus J (1980) Differential sensitivities of mammalian nerve fibers to local anesthetic agents. Anesthesiology 53: 467

44. Brown DT, Wildsmith JA Covino BG, Scott DB (1980) Effect of baricity on spinal anaesthesia with amethocaine. Br J Anaesth 52: 589

45. Chambers WA, Edström HH, Scott DB (1981) Effect of baricity on spinal anaesthesia with bupivacaine. Br J Anaesth 53: 279

46. Stephen GW, Lees MM, Scott DB (1969) Cardiovascular effects of epidural block combined with general anaesthesia. Br J Anaesth 41: 933

47. Steinbrook RA (1989) Respiratory effects of spinal anesthesia. Int Anesthesiol Clin 27: 40

48. Catenacci AJ, Sampathachar KR (1969) Ventilatory studies in obese patients during spinal anesthesia. Anesth Analg 48: 48

49. Greene NM (1981) Physiology of Spinal Anesthesia, 3rd ed. Baltimore: Williams & Wilkins p. 45

50. Steinbrook RA, Concepcion M, Topulos GP (1988) Ventilatory responses to hypercapnia during bupivacaine spinal anesthesia. Anesth Analg 67: 247

51. Steinbrook RA, Topulos GP, Concepcion M (1988) Ventilatory responses to hypercapnia during tetracaine spinal anesthesia. J Clin Anesth 1: 75

52. Pitkanen MT (1987) Body mass and spread of spinal anesthesia with bupivacaine. Anesth Analg 66:127

53. Giesecke AH Jr, Cale JO, Jenkins MT (1968) The prostate, ventilation, and anesthesia. JAMA 203: 389

54. Muravchick S, Johnson R (1986) Oxygenation of peripheral tissues in young and elderly patients during spinal anesthesia. Reg Anesth 11: 7

55. Davies MJ, Scott DA, Cook PT (1987) Continuous monitoring of arterial oxygen saturation with pulse oxymetry during spinal anesthesia. Reg Anesth 12: 63

56. Caplan R, Ward RJ, Posner K, Cheney FW (1988) Unexpected cardiac arrest during spinal anesthesia: a closed claims analysis of predisposing factors. Anesthesiology 68: 5

Chapter 3

Pharmacological considerations

Mechanism of action of local anaesthetics

The conduction of impulses along nerve fibres is due to changes in the electrical gradient across the nerve membrane. This results from the movement of ions, particularly sodium and potassium, across the membrane (Fig. 3.1). An adequate stimulus that reduces the resting membrane potential from approximately -90 mV to approximately -60 mV (the threshold potential level) produces a spontaneous rapid phase of depolarization (action potential). Depolarization in one segment of an unmyelinated nerve propagates to adjacent segments because of the difference in electrical potential between the depolarized and polarized areas (Fig. 3.2). In this way, an action potential generated by a stimulus applied to one end of a nerve travels along its entire length. In myelinated nerves the impulse jumps from one node of Ranvier to the next adjacent node (saltatory conduction). Repolarization returns the nerve membrane potential to the original resting level.

Fig. 3.1a. Resting state. Nerve fibre fully polarized with excess of Na ions (green) outside, and K ions (blue) inside, the membrane.

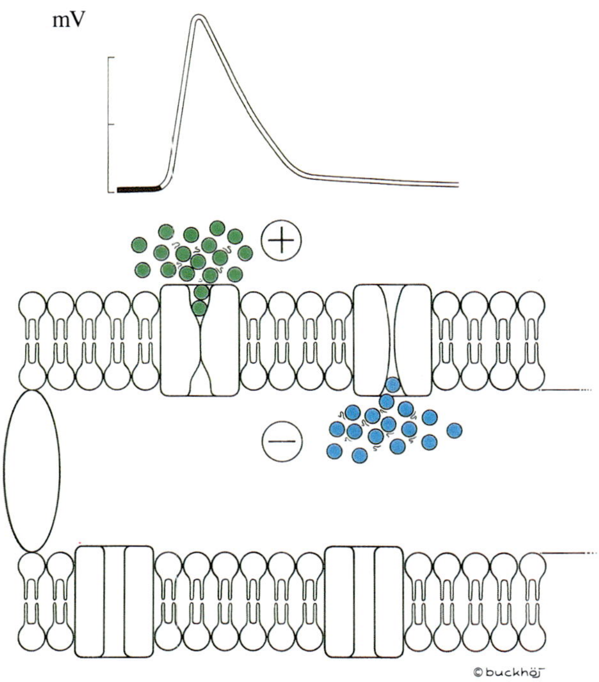

Fig. 3.1b. Depolarization due to inward movement of Na ions.

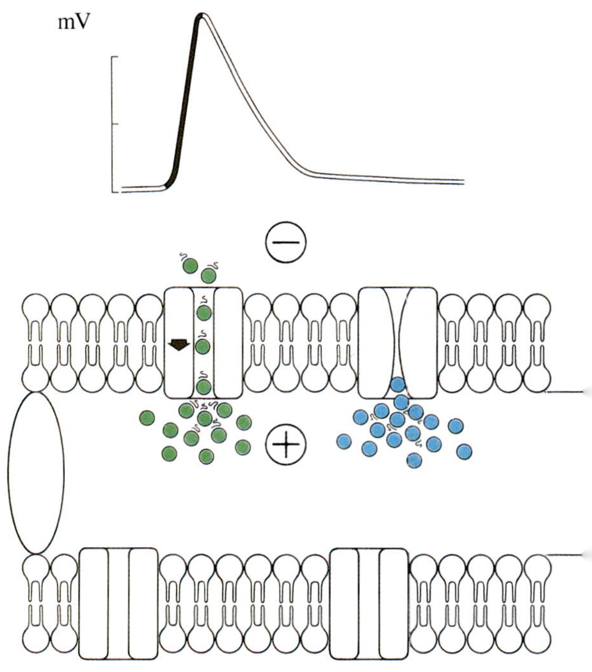

Depolarization is due to the inward passage of sodium ions from the extracellular to the intracellular space via specific sodium channels in the membrane (Fig. 3.1b). The flow of potassium ions from the interior to the exterior of the nerve causes repolarization (Fig. 3.1c). At the completion of the action potential, ionic equilibrium is re-established by the activation of the membrane sodium-potassium pump (Fig. 3.1d). Local anaesthetic agents prevent depolarization of the nerve membrane by blocking the flow of sodium ions.[1] Direct measurements of sodium and potassium conductance in the giant squid axon by voltage clamp techniques show that conventional local anaesthetics primarily block sodium currents with little effect on potassium currents.

Fig. 3.1c. Repolarization due to outward movement of K ions.

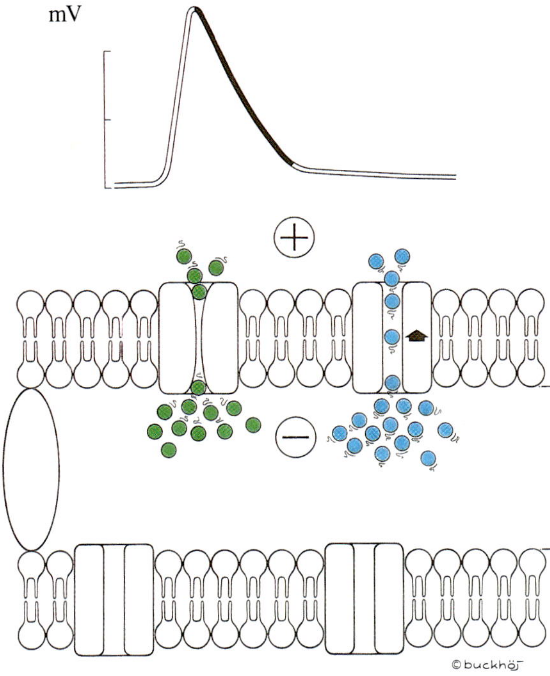

Fig. 3.1d. Nerve fibre fully polarized. Sodium-potassium pump restoring ions to the original disposition.

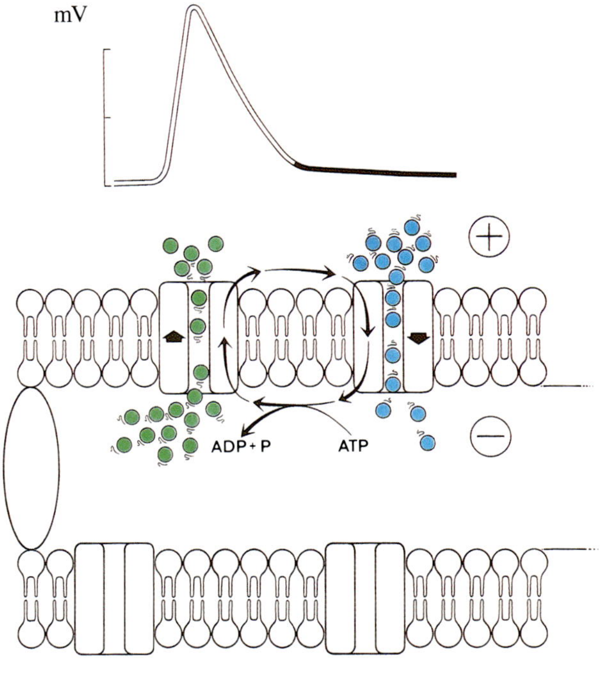

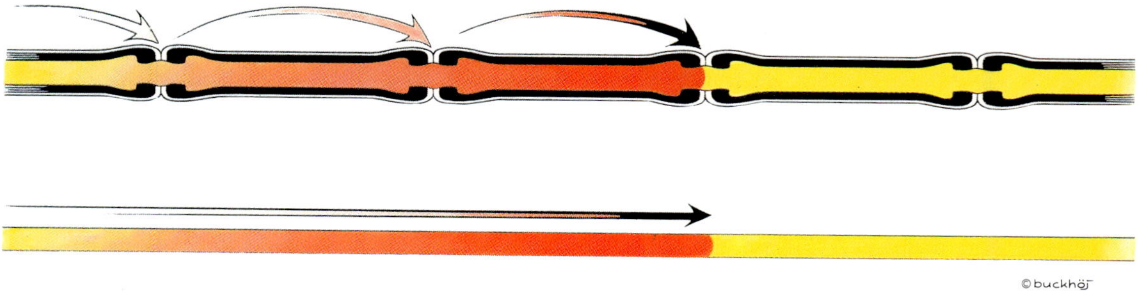

Fig. 3.2. a. and b. Propagation of a nerve impulse along myelinated and unmyelinated nerve fibres.
a. Impulse jumps from one node of Ranvier to the next in myelinated nerve fibres.
b. Impulse passes along the entire length of unmyelinated nerves.

The site of action of local anaesthetic agents undoubtedly involves the sodium channel in the nerve membrane (Fig. 3.3).

Fig. 3.3. Diagram of the structure of the nerve membrane which consists of a lipid bilayer and protein molecules which contain the sodium channels.

1. Lipid bilayer
2. Protein molecule
3. Sodium channel

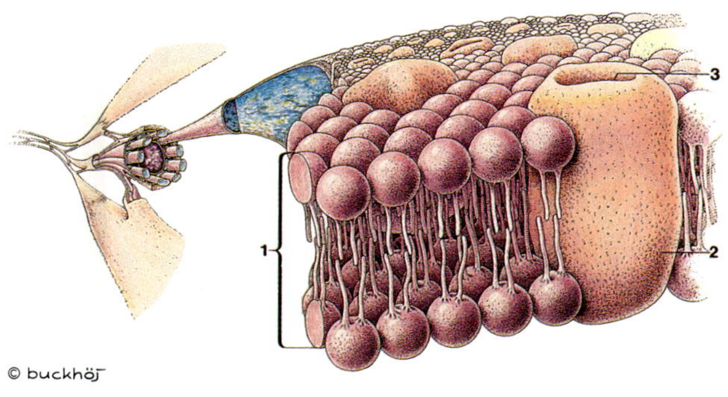

Local anaesthetics, such as lidocaine apparently penetrate the lipoprotein membrane matrix to reach the axoplasm and then enter the sodium channel where they probably interact with a specific receptor (Fig. 3.4).

Fig. 3.4. Passage of local anaesthetic molecules across the nerve membrane and entering a sodium channel from the axoplasmic surface.

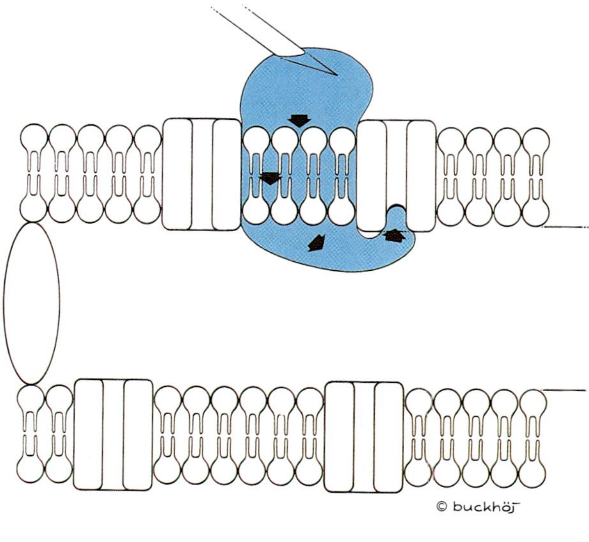

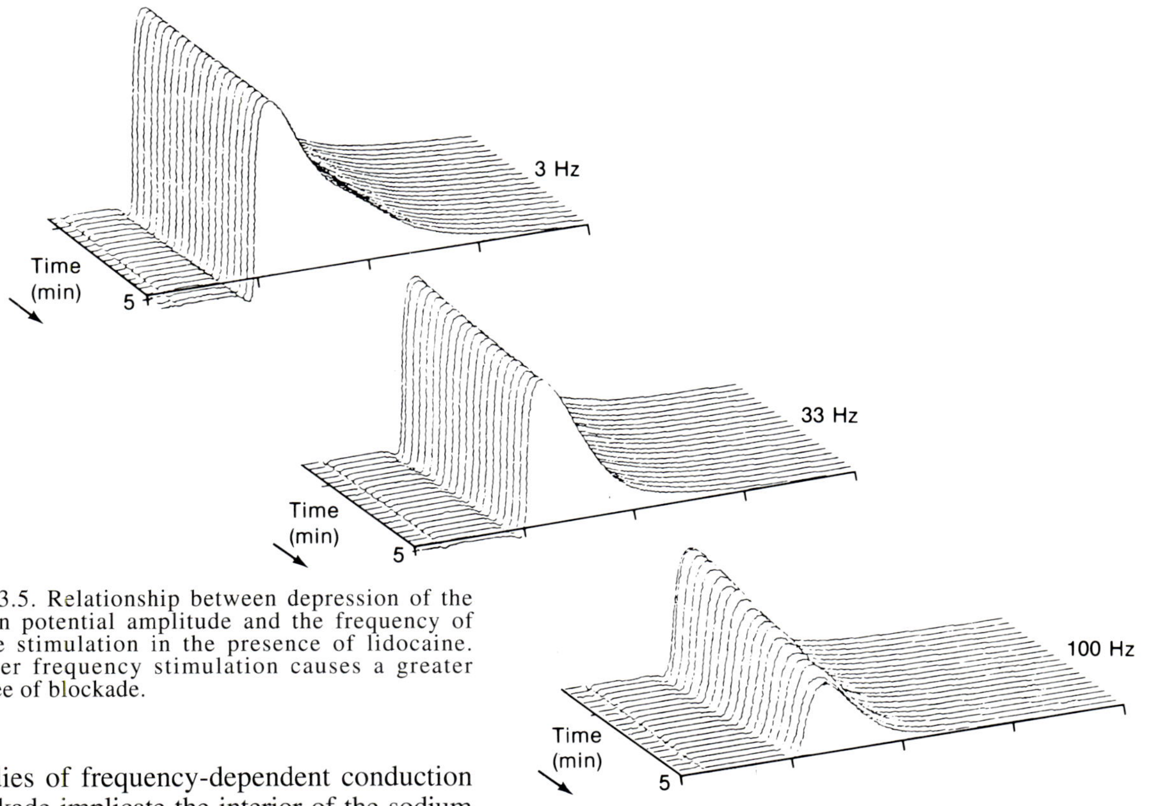

Fig. 3.5. Relationship between depression of the action potential amplitude and the frequency of nerve stimulation in the presence of lidocaine. Higher frequency stimulation causes a greater degree of blockade.

Studies of frequency-dependent conduction blockade implicate the interior of the sodium channel as the binding site for local anaesthetics.[2] For example, the amount of action potential suppression with agents like lidocaine is directly related to the frequency of nerve stimulation (Fig. 3.5). This phenomenon relates to the time that the sodium channels are in an open state. The sodium channel exists in three states; closed, open and inactive (Fig. 3.6). At rest the channel is closed so that neither sodium ions nor drug molecules can enter it. Stimulation of the nerve opens the channel, allowing sodium ions to enter its interior. With completion of the depolarization phase, the channel passes through an inactive state before returning to the resting closed state. As the frequency of stimulation increases, the sodium channels remain in an open state for longer periods. Therefore, at higher stimulation frequencies, the local anaesthetic agent, which has diffused across the membrane into the axoplasm, has a greater opportunity to penetrate the interior of the sodium channel.

Fig. 3.6. Various states of the sodium channel. 1. closed. 2. open. 3. inactiv.

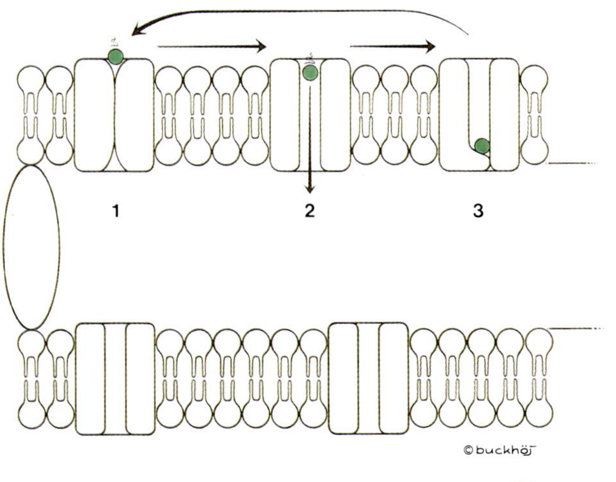

Diffusion of local anaesthetic across the nerve sheath and membrane to its site of action is an important aspect of nerve blockade and relates to the degree of ionization of the various drugs. In solution, local anaesthetic agents exist as uncharged molecules and as positively charged cations. The relative proportion of uncharged base to charged cation depends on the pKa of the specific local anaesthetic and the pH of the solution and is governed by the Henderson-Hasselbalch equation, i.e.

$$\mathrm{pH} = \mathrm{pKa} + \log \frac{[\text{base}]}{[\text{cation}]}$$

Since pKa is a constant, the relative proportion of free base and charged cation depends on the pH of the local anaesthetic solution. As the pH of the solution decreases, equilibrium shifts toward the charged cationic form and more cation is produced from free base. Conversely, as the pH increases, the equilibrium shifts toward the free base form. The uncharged base and the charged cationic form of the local anaesthetic are both important to the process of conduction blockade (Fig. 3.7). The base, but not the cationic form, diffuses readily through the nerve sheath and membrane into the axoplasm. In the axoplasm, a new equilibrium is established between base and cation and the charged cation binds to the receptor site in the sodium channel, inhibiting sodium conductance. Although the cation plays the major role in conduction blockade, the free base may also contribute by causing expansion of the nerve membrane, altering the sodium channel physically in such a way that sodium conductance is blocked.

Fig. 3.7. Diffusion of local anaesthetic agents across the nerve sheath and membrane to receptor sites in the sodium channel. Only the uncharged base form (LA) can cross the lipid membrane. When it reaches the axoplasm, ionization occurs and the charged cationic form (LAH^+) attaches to the receptor.

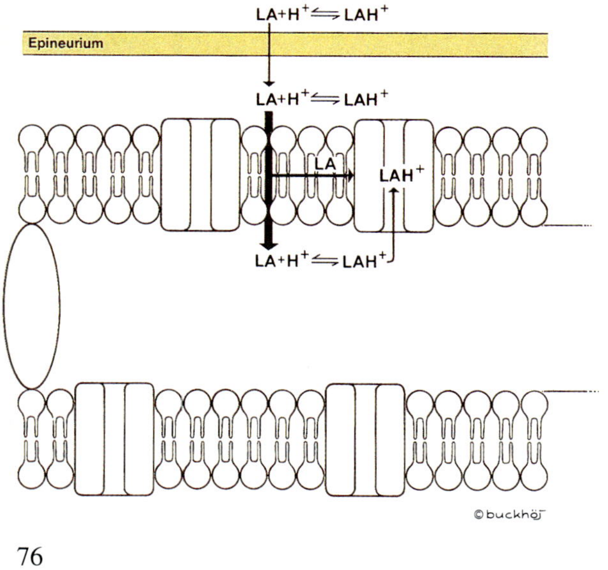

In summary, the sequence of events that results in conduction blockade in peripheral nerves by local anaesthetic agents is as follows:

1. Diffusion of the base form across the nerve sheath and membrane into the axoplasm
2. Re-equilibration between the base and cation in the axoplasm
3. Penetration of the cation into the sodium channel and attachment to a receptor site
4. Blockade of the sodium channel
5. Inhibition of sodium conductance
6. Decrease in the rate and degree of the depolarization phase of the action potential
7. Failure to achieve the threshold potential
8. Lack of development of a propagated action potential
9. Conduction blockade

Pharmacological basis of local anaesthetics

Chemical compounds that have local anaesthetic activity usually contain an aromatic group connected to an amine group by an intermediate chain. The clinically important local anaesthetics are divided into two distinct chemical groups (Table 3.1): amino-esters

Table 3.1. Chemical structure, physical-chemical properties, and pharmacological properties of local anaesthetic agents.

Agent	Structure (aromatic – chain – amine)	Physicochemical properties		Anesthetic profile		
		pKa	Octanol/buffer partition - coefficient*	Onset	Relative potency	Duration
Esters						
Procaine	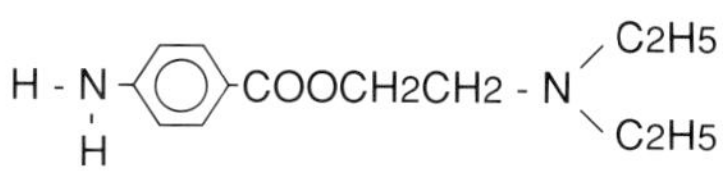	8.9	81	Slow	1	Short
Chloro-procaine	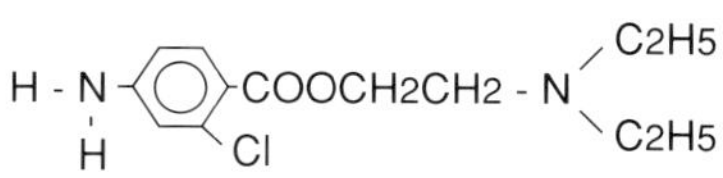	9.1	720	Fast	1	Short
Tetracaine	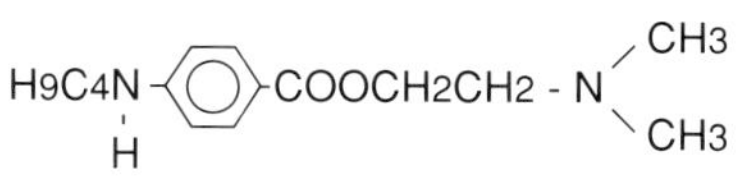	8.4	3615	Slow	8	Long
Amides						
Mepivacaine	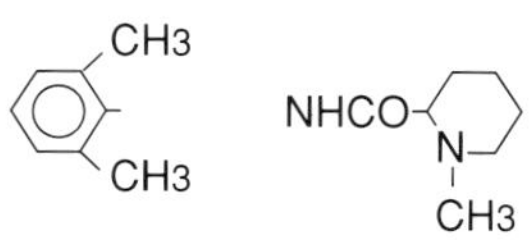	7.7	90	Fast	2	Moderate
Prilocaine	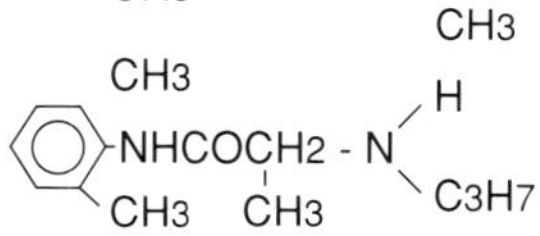	7.8	129	Fast	2	Moderate
Lidocaine	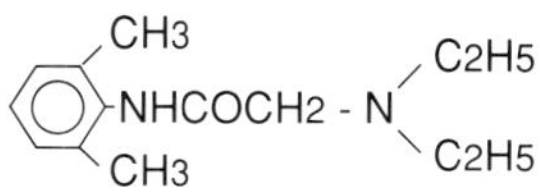	7.8	304	Fast	2	Moderate
Bupivacaine	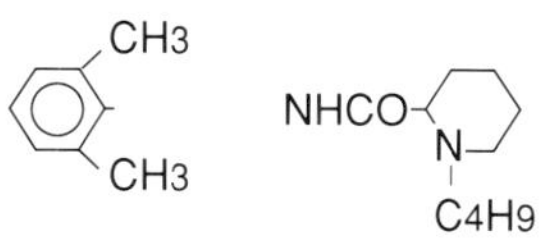	8.1	2565	Moderate	8	Long
Etidocaine	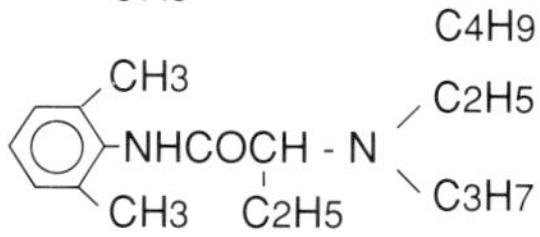	7.9	4900	Fast	6	Long

* Relative concentration (mol·L^{-1}) of uncharged local anaesthetic in octanol and buffer.

Local anaesthetics injected intrathecally bind to a greater extent in spinal nerve roots and the periphery of the spinal cord, i.e. where the small-diameter fibres are located.[6] Less drug diffuses into the dorsal root ganglion and centre of the spinal cord (Fig. 3.12). As a result, sensory anaesthesia occurs more rapidly than motor blockade. Ultimately sufficient drug reaches the large myelinated fibres to cause motor block.

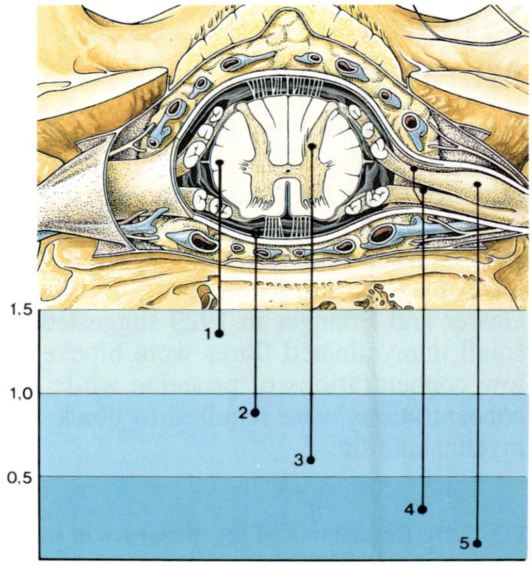

Fig. 3.12. Cross-section at T9 showing concentration of lidocaine in each structure following spinal administration at a lumbar interspace.

1. Periphery of spinal cord - 1.38 μg·mg^{-1}
2. CSF - 0,83 μg·mL^{-1}
3. Interior of spinal cord - 0.59 μg·mg^{-1}
4. Spinal roots - 0,32 μg·mg^{-1}
5. Dorsal root ganglion - 0,16 μg·mg^{-1}

Fig. 3.11. In vitro sensitivity of A, B and C fibres to various local anaesthetics.

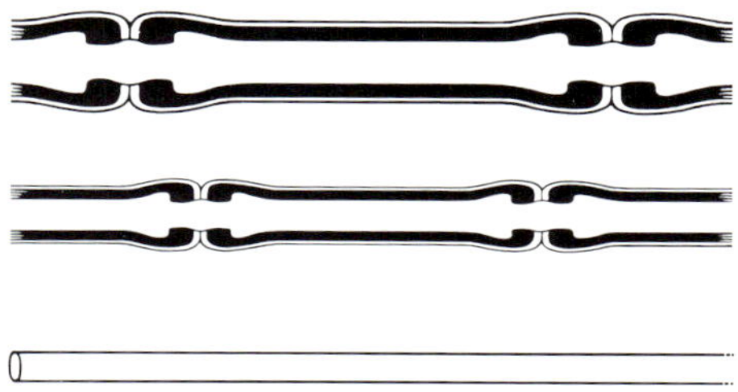

	Local anaesthetic concentration for conduction block (mmol· L^{-1})			
	Lidocaine	Tetracaine	Bupivacaine	Etidocaine
A- fibres	0,724	0,028	0,201	0,201
B- fibres	0,335	0,013	0,134	0,084
C- fibres	0,085	0,009	0,048	0,042

The amount of local anaesthetic used for spinal anaesthesia is an overdosage in relation to the minimum concentration required to block the various nerve fibre types and this is the reason for the relatively rapid blockade of sensory, sympathetic and motor fibres during clinical spinal anaesthesia. In general, the cephalad level of sympathetic blockade is approximately 2-3 segments higher than the level of sensory blockade, which, in turn, is higher than the level of motor block (Fig. 3.13). This differential level of nerve blockade may be related to several factors.

1. The anaesthetic concentration within the CSF declines as the cephalad distance from the site of injection increases.

2. In myelinated nerve fibres at least three consecutive nodes of Ranvier must be completely blocked to prevent conduction.

3. Decremental conduction block occurs when greater than three nodes are exposed to subminimal blocking concentrations of local anaesthetic.

The small B fibres in preganglionic sympathetic nerves possess short internodal distances (Fig. 3.10) and are most susceptible to conduction block, especially at upper spinal levels where CSF concentrations of local anaesthetic are low. The larger A-delta nociceptor fibres have longer internodal distances and require a higher local anaesthetic concentration for blockade. The larger motor A-alpha fibres have the greatest internodal distances and are blocked only when the local anaesthetic concentration is sufficient to inhibit three successive nodes.[7]

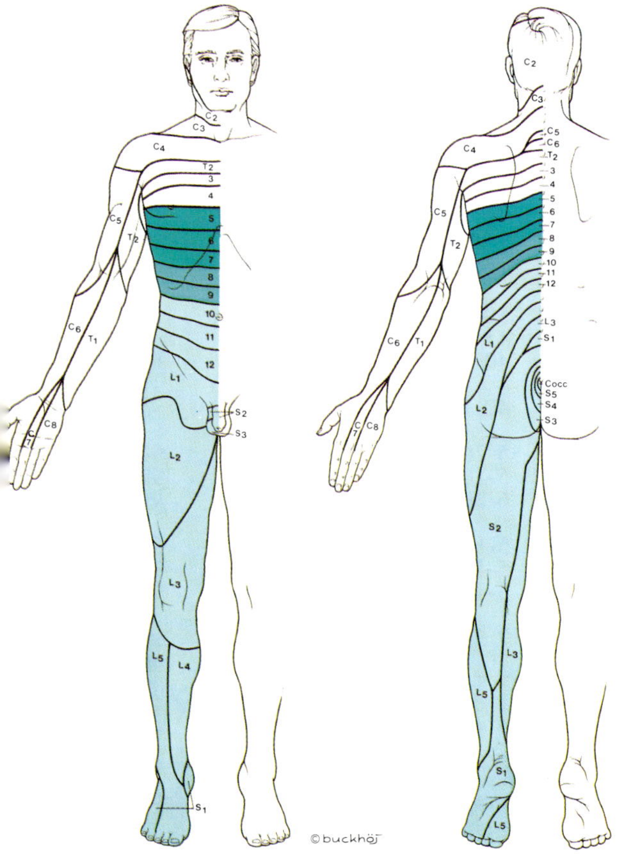

Fig. 3.13. Differential nerve block in spinal anaesthesia.

1. Sympathetic block to T5
2. Sensory block to T9
3. Motor block to T10

Differential sensory/motor blockade

Another important clinical consideration is the ability of local anaesthetic agents to cause a differential blockade of sensory and motor fibres. It is virtually impossible to produce spinal anaesthesia sufficient for surgery without impairment of motor function. However, the intrathecal administration of varying concentrations of procaine is used to produce a differential blockade of sensory, sympathetic, and motor fibres in the diagnosis of certain chronic pain syndromes. While bupivacaine shows a relative specificity for sensory fibres when employed for epidural blockade, it is impossible to separate sensory and motor blockade with subarachnoid administration. Nevertheless, bupivacaine causes a shorter duration of motor blockade than tetracaine folowing intrathecal administration (Fig. 3.15).[13]

Fig. 3.15. Duration of motor blockade after intrathecal bupivacaine and tetracaine.

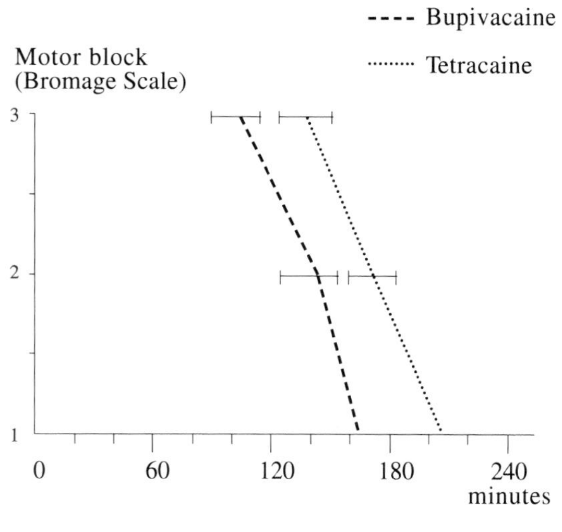

Factors influencing spinal anaesthetic activity

The factors that influence the spread and quality of spinal anaesthesia include:

1. The local anaesthetic drug.

2. The dosage of local anaesthetic.

3. The addition of a vasoconstrictor to the solution.

4. The baricity of the solution.

5. The addition of opioids to the local anaesthetic.

6. Pregnancy.

Local anaesthetic agents

The various agents may be classified as follows:

1. Agents of low anaesthetic potency and short duration of action, e.g. procaine

2. Agents of intermediate anaesthetic potency and duration of action, e.g. lidocaine and mepivacaine

3. Agents of high anaesthetic potency and prolonged duration of action, e.g. tetracaine, cinchocaine and bupivacaine.

Dosage of local anaesthetic agents

The mass of drug administered into the subarachnoid space will influence the onset, depth, duration and spread of anaesthesia. As the dose of local anaesthetic is increased, the frequency of satisfactory anaesthesia and the duration will increase while the onset time of anaesthesia will decrease. However, a linear relationship does not exist between the dose of local anaesthetic and the spread or duration. For example, increasing the dose of bupivacaine from 10 to 15 mg augments cephalad spread approximately four dermatomes and prolongs duration by approximately 60 min (Fig. 3.16).[14] However, a further increase in dose to 20 mg does not significantly increase either cephalad spread or duration. The dosage of local anaesthetic is the product of volume and concentration. No difference in depth, spread or duration of anaesthesia occurs with varying volumes and concentrations of bupivacaine when the dosage remains constant. For example, the spinal anaesthetic profile is similar when 15 mg of bupivacaine is administered either as 3 mL of 0.5% solution or as 2 mL of 0.75% solution.[14]

Fig. 3.16. Segmental spread of spinal anaesthesia with different doses of bupivacaine.

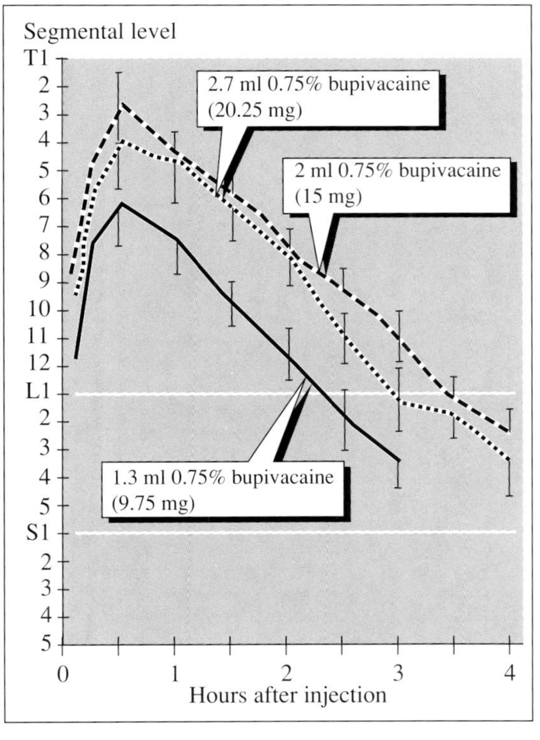

Addition of a vasoconstrictor to local anaesthetic solutions

Vasoconstrictors, particularly epinephrine and phenylephrine, are frequently added to local anaesthetic solutions to prolong the duration of spinal anaesthesia (Fig. 3.17).[15] These reportedly prolong the duration of tetracaine spinal anaesthesia by as little as 8% and as much as 100%.[16]

Results of studies on the effect of epinephrine on the blood levels of local anaesthetic administered intrathecally are conflicting. Some studies show a decrease in the blood levels when epinephrine is added to intrathecal lidocaine while others find no difference.[17,18] The prolongation of spinal anaesthesia by epinephrine may be due to a direct antinociceptive effect in the spinal cord. In this regard, clonidine, an alpha-adrenergic receptor agonist, produces analgesia following subarachnoid administration.[19]

Fig. 3.17. Effect of vasoconstrictors on the duration of spinal anaesthesia with tetracaine.

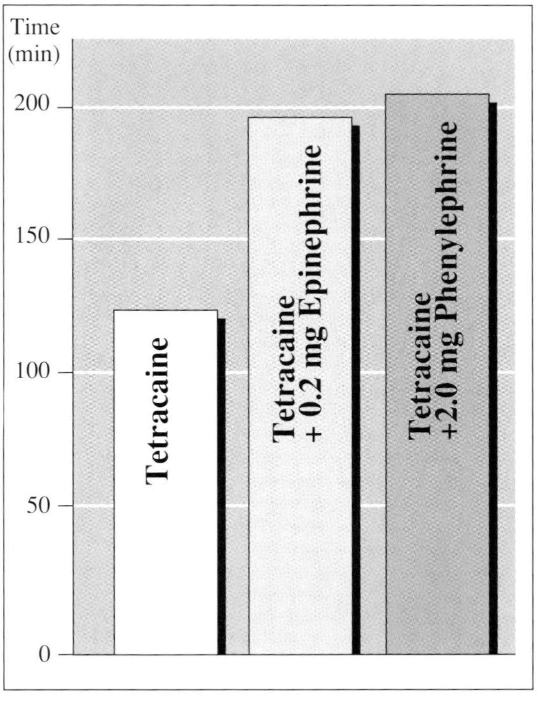

The doses of vasoconstrictor agents recommended for prolonging spinal anaesthesia are 0.2 to 0.3 mg of epinephrine and 2 to 5 mg of phenylephrine. However, there is no precise relationship between the dose of vasoconstrictors and the prolongation of anaesthesia and there is controversy concerning the amount of prolongation that can be expected. Considering the variability in the prolongation of spinal anaesthesia with these agents, there is little evidence to suggest that one agent has any advantage over the other.[15]

The ability of vasoconstrictor agents to prolong spinal anaesthesia may vary with the local anaesthetic agent used. For example, both epinephrine and phenylephrine significantly extend the duration of tetracaine at all dermatomal levels.[20] On the other hand, epinephrine and phenylephrine do not prolong two or four segment sensory regression of lidocaine or bupivacaine spinal anaesthesia (Fig. 3.18).[21,22] However, lower thoracic, lumbar and sacral anaesthesia is prolonged by vasoconstrictors added to solutions of lidocaine and bupivacaine. Therefore, the duration of spinal anaesthesia for lower extremity surgery can be prolonged by adding vasoconstrictors to tetracaine, bupivacaine and lidocaine.

Fig. 3.18. Effect of epinephrine on lidocaine spinal anaesthesia. Note the absence of dose response.

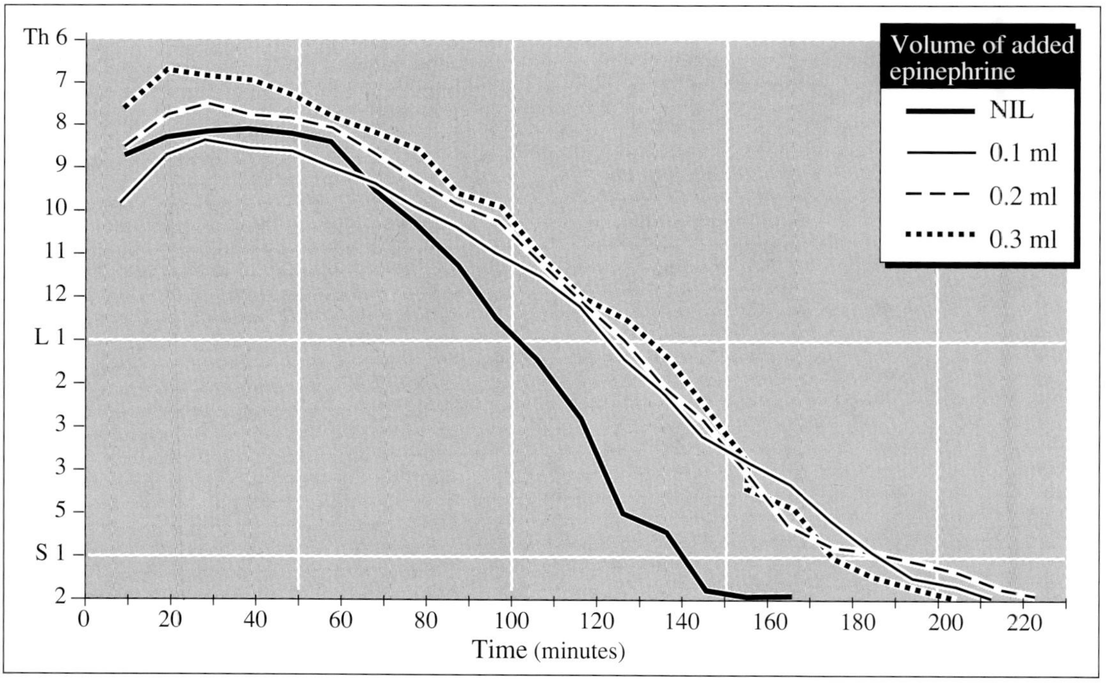

However, for abdominal operations, adding vasoconstrictors to lidocaine or bupivacaine may not prolong duration to the same extent as when they are added to tetracaine. The different effect of adding vasoconstrictors to tetracaine, bupivacaine and lidocaine may be due to changes in spinal cord and dural blood flow (Fig. 3.19).[23-25] Tetracaine markedly increases spinal cord and dural blood flow and this increase is inhibited by the addition of epinephrine. On the other hand, bupivacaine decreases spinal cord and dural blood flow and this is only slightly altered by the addition of epinephrine. Lidocaine is intermediate in its effect on spinal cord and dural blood flow.

Fig. 3.19. Effect of epinephrine on spinal cord and dural blood flow during spinal anaesthesia with lidocaine, bupivacaine and tetracaine (Adapted with permission from Kozody et al[23-25]).

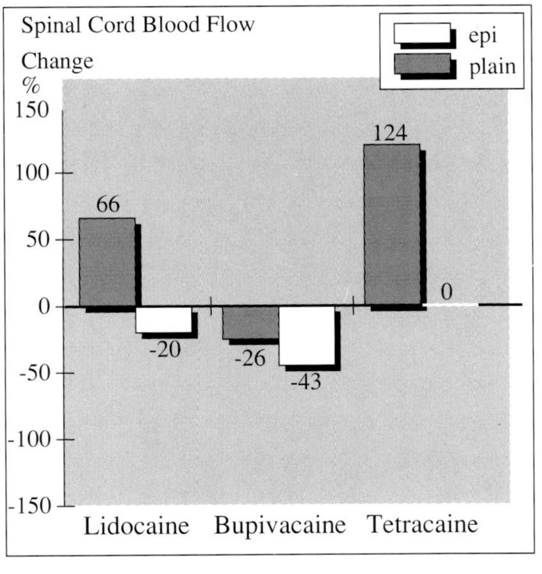

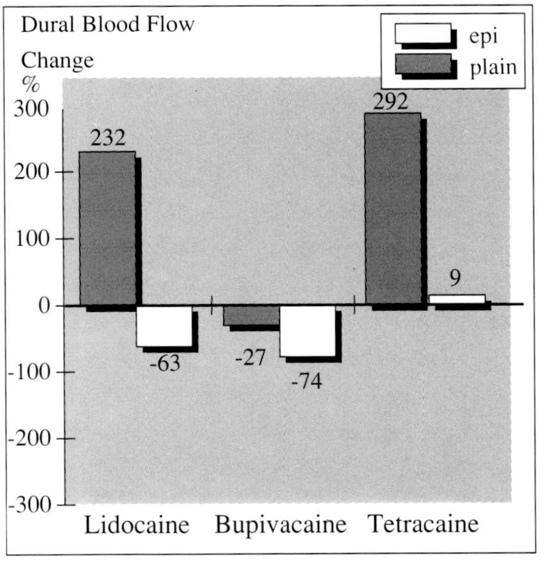

Baricity of local anaesthetic solutions

Local anaesthetics used for spinal anaesthesia are characterized according to their baricity (hypobaric, isobaric or hyperbaric). **Baricity** is the ratio of the density of a local anaesthetic solution at a specified temperature to the density of cerebrospinal fluid at the same temperature. **Density** is the weight in grams of 1 mL of a solution at a specified temperature. **Specific gravity** is the ratio of the density of a solution at a specified temperature to the density of water at the same temperature.

According to these definitions, an isobaric local anaesthetic solution has a baricity of 1 while hypobaric and hyperbaric solutions have baricities less than or greater than unity, respectively. It is important to note that density varies inversely with temperature. Therefore, a local anaesthetic which has the same density as cerebrospinal fluid at 37°C is more dense (hyperbaric) at room temperature (the temperature at which local anaesthetics are usually injected) than cerebrospinal fluid at 37°C.[26] However, the clinically important density of a local anaesthetic solution is that which is measured at 37°C because, during spinal anaesthesia, local anaesthetic solutions rapidly equilibrate with the temperature of cerebrospinal fluid.[27]

The density of normal human cerebrospinal fluid with 95% confidence limits at 37°C is 1.0001 - 1.0005. Therefore, local anaesthetic solutions with density less than 0.9998 (99.9% confidence limits) at 37°C will be hypobaric in any patient. Similarly, solutions at 37°C with density greater than 1.0008 (99.9% confidence limits) will be reliably hyperbaric in all patients (Fig. 3.20). Because of the variability in the density of cerebrospinal fluid it is difficult to predict that a solution will, in fact, be isobaric in all patients. Nevertheless, solutions with densities between 0.9998 and 1.0008 behave functionally as if they have the same density as cerebrospinal fluid.

Fig. 3.20. Effect of baricity on the diffusion of solution injected into the subarachnoid space in the upright position.

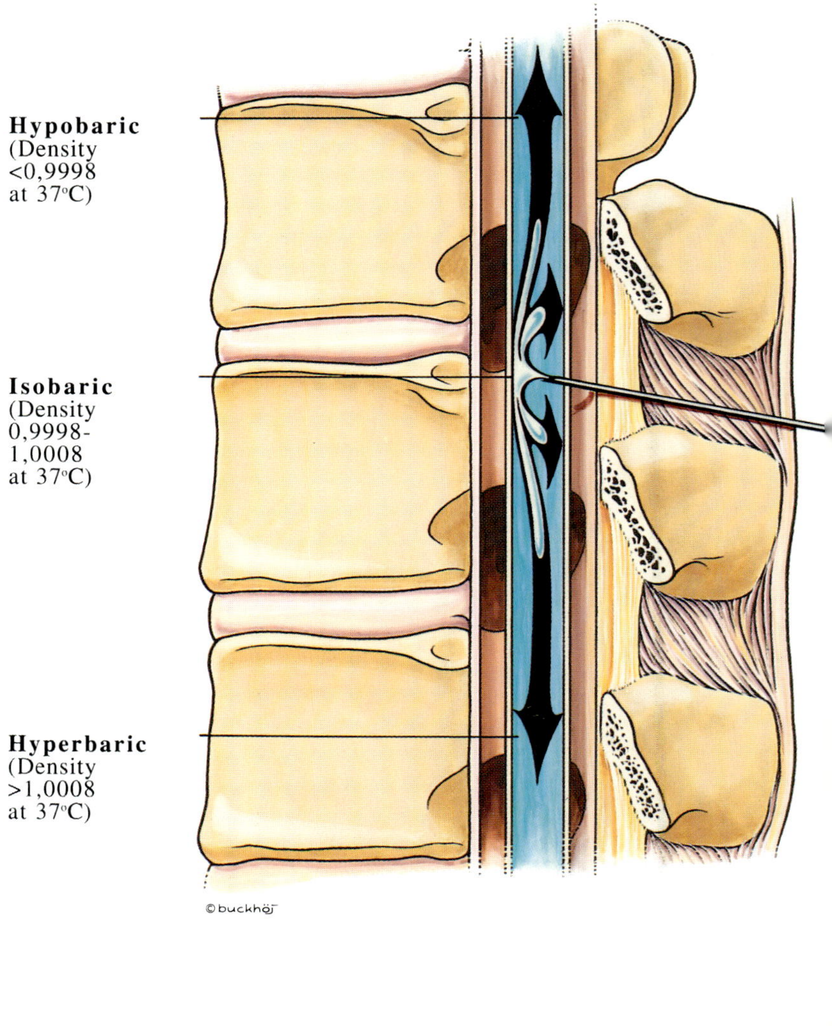

Local anaesthetic solutions used for spinal anaesthesia are formulated with water, normal saline or dextrose to make them hypobaric, isobaric or hyperbaric respectively (Table 3.3).

Table 3.3. Density and baricity of local anaesthetics commonly used for spinal anaesthesia. Ref Lambert DH, BG Covino, Hyperbaric, hypobaric and isobaric spinal anesthesia. Res Staff Phys, 1987 33:79.

Agent	Usual conc. (%)	Diluent	Density (37°C)	Baricity
CSF			1,0003	1,0000
Procaine	2,5	Distilled water	0,9986	0,9983
	10,0	None	1,0107	1,0104
Lidocaine	2,0	Normal saline	1,0007	1,0004
	5,0	7,5% Dextrose	1,0265	1,0262
Bupivacaine	0,5	Normal saline	0,9993	0,9990
	0,75	8,25% Dextrose	1,0230	1,0227
Tetracaine	<0,33	Distilled water	<0,9980	<0,0077
	0,5	Normal saline	1,0000	0,9997
	0,5	5,0% Dextrose	1,0136	1,0133
Cinchocaine	0,06	Normal saline	0,9967	0,9964
	0,5	Normal saline	0,9992	0,9990
	0,25	5,0% Dextrose	1,0111	1,0108

CSF density at 37°C (99,9% confidence limits) = 0,9998-1,0008.[26]

The significance of baricity lies in the fact that isobaric solutions tend to remain in the area where they are injected into the CSF, while hypobaric solutions "float" upwards and hyperbaric solutions "sink"(Fig. 3.20). Therefore, it is possible, by selecting the appropriate baricity and patient position (Fig. 3.21), to "direct" the local anaesthetic to nerves that need to be anaesthetized. For example, it is possible to anaesthetize the sacral nerves by injecting a hyperbaric solution with the patient in the upright position or a hypobaric solution with the patient in the prone jack-knife position.

Fig. 3.21. The effect of position and baricity on the distribution of a local anaesthetic solution in the spinal subarachnoid space. The tubular figures represent the dural sac with CSF. The black areas show the local anaesthetic solution.

A. Upright position for saddle block. A hyperbaric solution, "sinks" to the most dependent area.

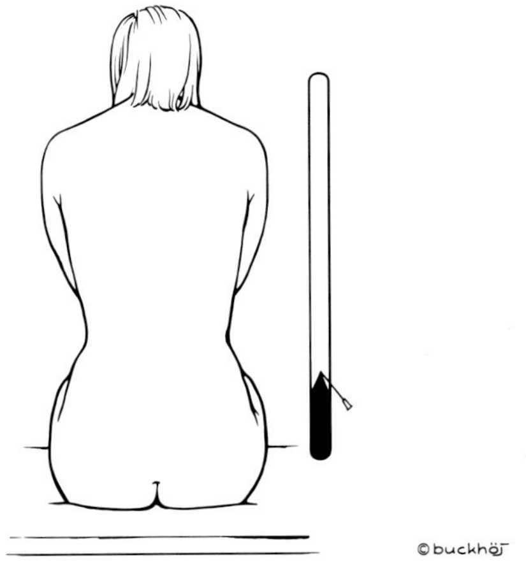

B. Prone jack-knife position for rectal surgery. A hypobaric solution, "floats" to the upper most area.

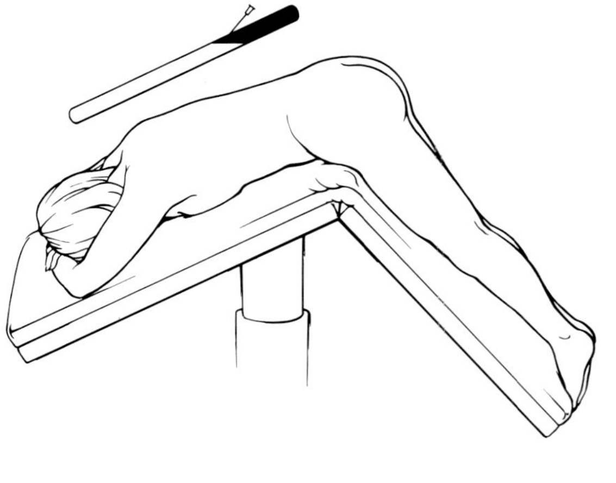

In the supine horizontal posture, when spread is least affected by gravity, hyperbaric solutions nevertheless show the greatest spread and the shortest duration of anaesthesia.[28] Conversely, hypobaric solutions have the least cephalad spread, but the longest duration (Fig. 3.22). Isobaric solutions are intermediate in terms of cephalad spread and duration of anaesthesia. Baricity also affects the degree of motor block. Isobaric solutions of bupivacaine produce more motor blockade than hyperbaric solutions, because the dose per spinal nerve is greater when cephalad spread is restricted. Perhaps the greatest difference between solutions of different baricity is the variability in spread. Hyperbaric solutions show the least variation in cephalad spread while isobaric and hypobaric solutions show the most (Fig. 3.23).[28]

Addition of opioids to local anaesthetics

Opioids added to local anaesthetic solutions increase the degree and duration of analgesia when injected into the subarachnoid space (see p. 98).

Fig. 3.22 Mean of the maximum heights of analgesia produced by different specific gravities of tetracaine. Reproduced with permission Brown et al[28]

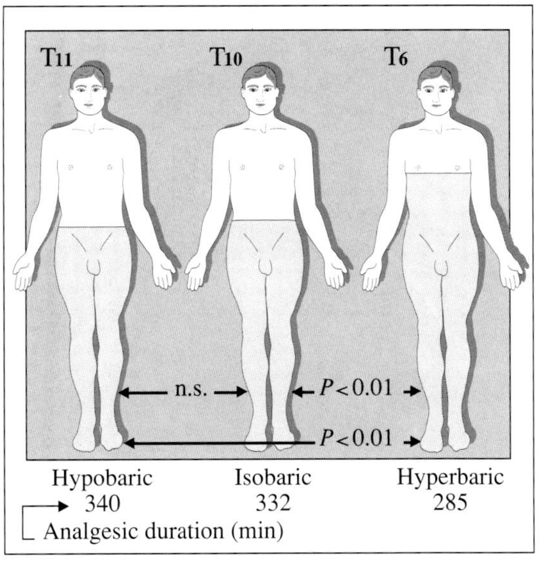

Fig. 3.23. Individual maximum height (right and left) of analgesia 15 min. after the injection of either 10 or 15 mg of tetracaine. Note greater consistency of the hyperbaric solution. Reproduced with permission Brown et al[28]

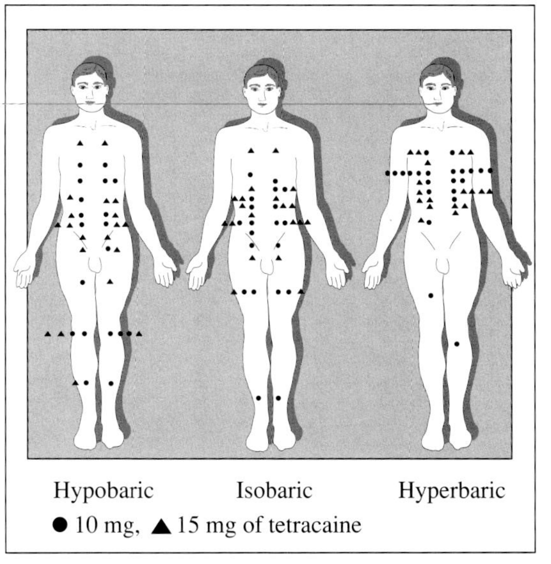

The vascular absorption of intrathecally administered local anaesthetics may also be related to baricity. The peak plasma levels of lidocaine and bupivacaine occur more rapidly after administration of hyperbaric solutions compared to isobaric solutions (Fig. 3.27).[34] However, there is no significant difference in the maximum plasma concentrations achieved with these solutions. The more rapid vascular absorption of hyperbaric solutions may be related to the greater spread of these solutions within the subarachnoid space, and the greater surface area available for diffusion and absorption. Since the total dosage employed for spinal anaesthesia is extremely small, the peak plasma concentrations are so low that systemic toxic effects will not occur.

Spinal anaesthesia itself may alter the rate of tissue redistribution and elimination of local anaesthetic agents. The sympathetic blockade, due to spinal anaesthesia, decreases hepatic blood flow and alters the vascular perfusion of various tissue beds, which may lead to decreased metabolism and elimination. On the other hand, the blood concentrations of local anaesthetics following subarachnoid administration are so low that these changes in distribution and elimination are of little practical significance.

Fig. 3.26. Mean ± SE venous plasma levels of lidocaine following epidural or subarachnoid administration of 75 mg. Bar graph shows mean ± SE maximum venous plasma levels of lidocaine following epidural or subarachnoid administration * $p < 0.05$; ** $p < 0.01$. Reproduced with permission, Giasi et al.[35]

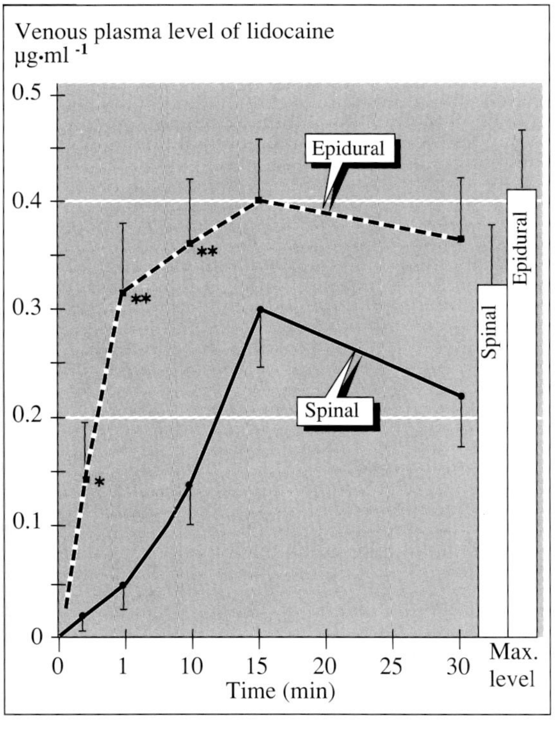

Fig. 3.27. Mean ± SE venous plasma concentrations of bupivacaine obtained after subarachnoid administration of 15 mg. Note more rapid absorption with the hyperbaric solution. Reproduced with permission, Burm[34]

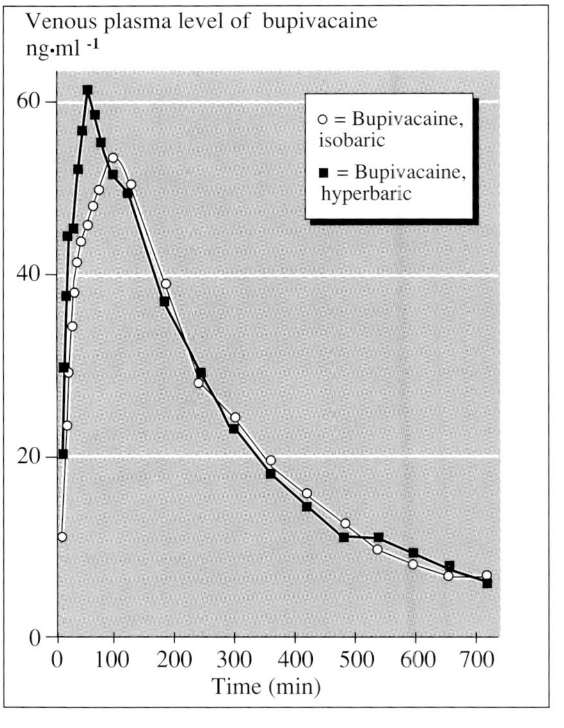

Specific spinal anaesthetic agents

(See Table 3.2, p. 84)

Procaine

This agent, the first synthetic compound to be employed for regional anaesthesia, is still used as a 10% solution (pH 5.4). This solution, without dextrose, is hyperbaric due to the high concentration of procaine. Procaine produces spinal anaesthesia of 30-60 min duration. The usual dose is 100-200 mg (1-2 mL). Procaine is also used diagnostically for differential subarachnoid blockade in patients with various pain syndromes.

Tetracaine

Synthesized in 1931, tetracaine is a potent local anaesthetic and continues to be widely used for spinal anaesthesia. The onset of spinal anaesthesia occurs in 5-10 min and usually persists for 2-3 h, but may last 6-8 h even without a vasoconstrictor. Tetracaine is available as a 1% solution (pH 3-4) or as easily soluble (niphanoid) crystals. Hyperbaric and isobaric solutions of 0.5% tetracaine are prepared by mixing the 1% solution with equal volumes of either 10% dextrose or 0.9% saline, respectively. Hypobaric solutions are prepared by mixing 1 mL of tetracaine with 4-9 mL of sterile water, producing a final anaesthetic concentration of 0.2-0.1%. The usual dose of tetracaine varies from 5-20 mg. Vasoconstrictors may significantly increase the duration of anaesthesia produced by tetracaine.

Lidocaine

Lidocaine, the first amino-amide local anaesthetic agent, was synthesized in 1943. Lidocaine is most commonly used for spinal anaesthesia as a hyperbaric 5% solution containing 7.5% dextrose. The pH of this solution is approximately 6.5. A hyperbaric solution of 1.5% lidocaine with 7.5% dextrose is also available for spinal anaesthesia in some countries. Lidocaine (2%) without dextrose has also been used for spinal anaesthesia. This solution is considered to be isobaric. Hyperbaric solutions of 5% lidocaine cause profound sensory anaesthesia and motor block within 5 min. The usual dose is 40-100 mg, which will provide a duration of approximately 45-90 min.

Mepivacaine

A hyperbaric 4% solution of mepivacaine with 9% dextrose is commercially available in some European countries. The usual dose is 40-100 mg and this will produce rapid and profound sensory anaesthesia with a duration similar to that of hyperbaric 5% lidocaine.

Bupivacaine

Bupivacaine is the most recent drug to be introduced specifically for spinal anaesthesia. It is available in various countries either as a 0.75% hyperbaric solution with 8.25% dextrose or as a 0.5% hyperbaric solution with 8.0% dextrose. The pH of these solutions is approximately 5.5. Isobaric (plain) solutions of 0.5% and 0.75% bupivacaine are also available. The usual dose of either isobaric or hyperbaric bupivacaine is 7.5-22.5 mg. Sensory anaesthesia is usually complete within 10 min and persists for approximately 2-3 h. The addition of a vasoconstrictor to bupivacaine solutions has less effect on the duration of anaesthesia than is the case with tetracaine.

Cinchocaine (dibucaine)

Cinchocaine is a quinolone derivative with an amide link in the molecule. It is the most potent of the spinal anaesthetic agents. Concentrations of 0.25% cinchocaine provide anaesthesia similar to 0.5% tetracaine. It is available in various countries as 0.067% (hypobaric), 0.5% (isobaric) and 0.25% or 0.5% (hyperbaric) solutions. This once popular agent is no longer commercially available in most countries.

Table 3.4. Classification of opioid receptor subtypes.

Mu_1	Mu_2	Delta	Kappa	Sigma
Analgesia: somatic visceral Miosis	Apnoea Bradycardia Dependency Euphoria	Modulate Mu receptors	Analgesia: visceral Sedation	Dysphoria Mydriasis Tachycardia Tachypnoea

Intrathecal opioids

The subarachnoid administration of opioids is used to potentiate spinal analgesia and relieve pain, particularly postoperative pain.[36] Specific opioid receptors (Table 3.4) are present in the ventromedial medulla, the periaqueductal area of the brain and in the substantia gelatinosa of the spinal cord.[37] The various effects of opioids are believed to be mediated by the several receptor subtypes.[38] "Mu" receptors are activated by morphine-type agonists, resulting in analgesia, miosis and respiratory depression. "Delta" receptors interact with d-ala-d-leu-enkephalin (DADL) and modulate Mu receptor activity. "Kappa" receptors interact with ketocyclazocine and related benzomorphan compounds, which cause visceral analgesia but less respiratory depression compared to Mu receptor agonists. "Sigma" receptors, which are activated by SKF-10,047, are not involved in analgesia but do produce excitation and dysphoria.

Mu receptors are subdivided into two groups - Mu_1 mediating analgesia and Mu_2 causing respiratory depression. This classification implies that a Mu_1 agonist could provide analgesia without respiratory depression. Currently, no drug specific for Mu_1 receptors is available. The so-called mixed agonist/antagonists (e.g. butorphanol, nalbuphine) produce analgesia by interacting with kappa receptors. Endogenous and exogenous opioids produce analgesia by interacting directly with receptors at spinal and supraspinal levels and also produce analgesia indirectly by activating descending antinociceptive pathways (see p. 56).

Table 3.5. Opioid peptides and precursors.

Precursor	Peptide	Structure
Proenkephalin	Met-enkephalin Leu-enkephalin	Tyr-Gly-Gly-Phe-Met Tyr-Gly-Gly-Phe-Leu
Pro-opiomelanocortin	Beta-endorphin	Tyr-Gly-Gly-Phe-Met-Thr-Ser-Glu-Lys-Ser-Glu-Thr-Pro-Leu-Val-Thr-Leu-Phe-Lys-Asp-Ala-Ile-Ile-Lys-Asp-Ala-His-Lys-Lys-Gly-Glu
Prodynorphin	Dynorphin	Tyr-Gly-Gly-Phe-Leu-Arg-Arg-Ile

Endogenous opioid peptides

The term "endorphin" is used generically to denote all endogenous opioid peptides. There are a number of these involved in the modulation of pain transmission, the most important being met-enkephalin, leu-enkephalin, beta-endorphin and dynorphin. The two enkephalins each consist of 5 amino acids, the first four of which are identical (tyrosine-glycine-glycine-phenylalanine). Methionine added to this sequence produces met-enkephalin while the addition of leucine produces leu-enkephalin. Pro-opiomelanocortin (pro-ACTH-endorphin) gives rise to beta-endorphin, a 31 amino acid residue that begins with the met-enkephalin sequence. Prodynorphin is the precursor to dynorphin, a peptide that begins with the leu-enkephalin sequence (Table 3.5).

The activity of endorphins is due to their tyramine-like structure.[39] The opioid receptor is postulated to contain a "T"-site that binds the tyrosine residue of the enkephalins, a "P"-site that binds the phenylalanine residue of the enkephalins and an "N"-site that binds nitrogen ion (Fig. 3.28). The enkephalins therefore bind to the T-, P- and N-sites, while morphine interacts only with the T- and N-sites, and meperidine only with the P- and N-sites. Because all of the endorphins begin with the same amino acid sequence (Tyr-Gly-Gly-Phe), their differing effects are due to the unique amino acid sequence beyond this chain (Table 3.5).

Fig. 3.28. Interaction of the opioid receptor with enkephalin, morphine and pethidine. The opioid receptor contains T-, N- and P- sites. The T-site preferentially binds hydroxylated aromatic rings similar to that which occurs in tyrosine. The P-site preferentially binds non-hydroxylated rings similar to the one found in phenylalanine, and the anionic N-site binds nitrogen groups. Adapted with permission, Thorpe[39]

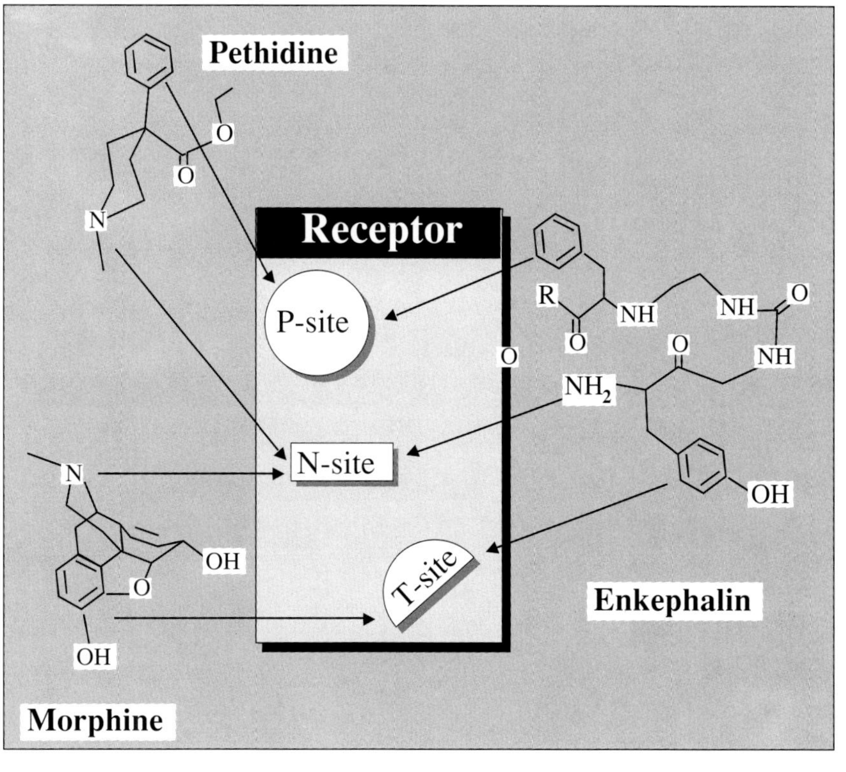

Clinical aspects of intrathecal opioids

Opioids, like local anaesthetics, can be classified on the basis of pKa and lipid solubility (partition coefficient) (Table 3.6). On injection into the CSF, opioids distribute themselves between nerve tissue and CSF on the basis of their partition coefficient. Thus, morphine, which has a low partition coefficient, remains within the CSF in substantial quantity and diffuses slowly into nerve tissue, accounting for its delayed onset and prolonged duration of effect. In addition, it is able to migrate cephalad with the possibility of reaching the brainstem respiratory centre, causing respiratory depression. On the other hand, it has the advantage of extending the spread of analgesia well beyond the site of injection. The other opioids are all much more lipid soluble than morphine and remain in the CSF for shorter periods. Therefore, onset is more rapid and duration shorter. These agents are much less likely to migrate rostrally and while respiratory depression is therefore unlikely, they must be injected near to the required site of action to be effected.

Table 3.6. Physicochemical properties of opioids.

Opioid	Molecular weight	pKa	Partition coefficient
Morphine	285	7.9	1.42
Pethidine	247	8.5	38.8
Methadone	309	9.3	116
Fentanyl	336	8.4	813
Sufentanil	386	8.0	1778

Intrathecal opioids are not as widely used as those given epidurally, and are usually administered by a single injection because spinal catheters are not often continued postoperatively. However, the intrathecal route offers many advantages: faster onset, better efficacy, lower blood levels and decreased side-effects. Intrathecal opioids are particularly useful in chronic pain states where implantable devices benefit from the use of low volumes. On the other hand epidural catheters have been left in place for prolonged periods without sequelae and the epidural route is the most popular for administering multiple doses of opioids during labour and for postoperative pain management.

Fig. 3.29. Prolongation of analgesia after Caesarean section by adding fentanyl to bupivacaine. Reproduced with permission, Hunt et al[40]

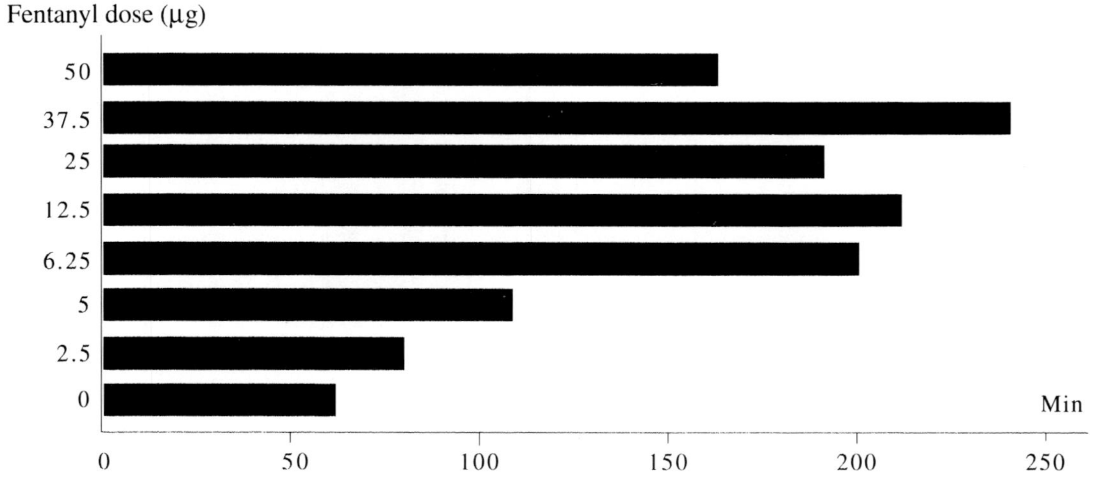

The addition of opioids to intrathecal local anaesthetics improves both the quality and the duration of postoperative analgesia. 6.25 to 50 μg of fentanyl added to bupivacaine spinal anaesthesia produces approximately 2-4 h of postoperative analgesia in Caesarean section patients (Fig. 3.29). However, doses in excess of 6.25 μg of fentanyl are unnecessary because the duration of analgesia is not further prolonged while the incidence of side- effects increases.[40] The addition of 0.1-0.25 mg of morphine to bupivacaine similarly improves the quality of spinal analgesia and results in 12-24 h postoperative analgesia[41,42] without depressing the ventilatory response to carbon dioxide.[42] Sufentanil has also been used but has no advantage over fentanyl.

The improvement in the quality of analgesia apparently results from the action of the opioid in the substantia gelatinosa. Thus, a synergistic analgesic effect occurs between the opioid (inhibiting pain transmission in the dorsal horn) and the local anaesthetic (blocking conduction in the nerve roots and spinal cord). Analgesia is, therefore, improved because two distinct mechanisms interrupt the pain pathway.

The major concern with the use of intrathecal or epidural opioids (particularly morphine) is the occurrence of late respiratory depression. This effect is dose related. The initial studies and case reports of intrathecal morphine included excessive doses (e.g. up to 20 mg), and it is not surprising that potentially lethal respiratory depression occurred. As a result, intrathecal opioids are less popular than epidural opioids. However, morphine injected epidurally must diffuse through the dura into the CSF to reach the dorsal horn. Since the usual epidural dose of morphine is 5 mg, an appropriate intrathecal dose is in the order of 0.2-0.5 mg. Doses of intrathecal morphine in the range of 0.06-0.3 mg produce approximately 20-24 h of analgesia in 60-70% of patients.[43-45] Higher doses of intrathecal morphine provide analgesia in 100% of patients at the expense of higher incidences of respiratory depression (Fig. 3.30).[46] Naloxone is effective in reversing respiratory depression, but may require prolonged administration, e.g. by infusion.

Nausea, vomiting, pruritus and urinary retention are the most common side-effects seen with spinally administered opioids.[47] These side-effects may be treated with small doses of intravenous naloxone without antagonizing analgesia.[48]

Fig. 3.30. Effect of increasing doses of intrathecal morphine on postoperative analgesia and respiratory depression. Adapted from refs 43-46.

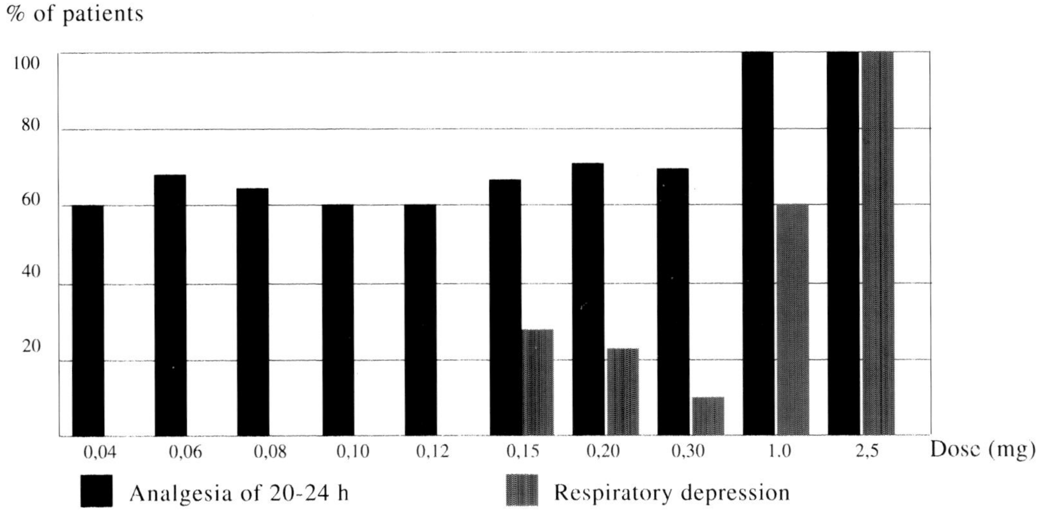

The dura is made chiefly of collagen fibres and some elastic fibres (Fig. 1.12, p. 20). The collagen fibres are orientated in diverse directions while the elastic fibres generally run longitudinally.[5]

The dura is also variable in its thickness (0.5 to 2 mm) even in the same individual. The thicker it is, the greater the retraction of the hole. The typical "tin-lid" hole is produced by all needle tips with a cutting edge.[4] When a non-cutting needle is used or when a cutting needle is inserted with the point parallel to the longitudinal fibres, an ellipsoidal hole is produced (Fig. 4.4), compared to a more round hole when the needle tip is at right angles to the fibres.[4,6]

Fig. 4.4. Scanning electron micrograph of dural puncture hole made with a 25 G Whitacre (non-cutting) needle. Viewed from intrathecal side of dura. Note "ellipsoidal" configuration and the torn rather than cut dural fibres. (Photos courtesy of Drs. Mark Johnson and Vladimer Bittner).

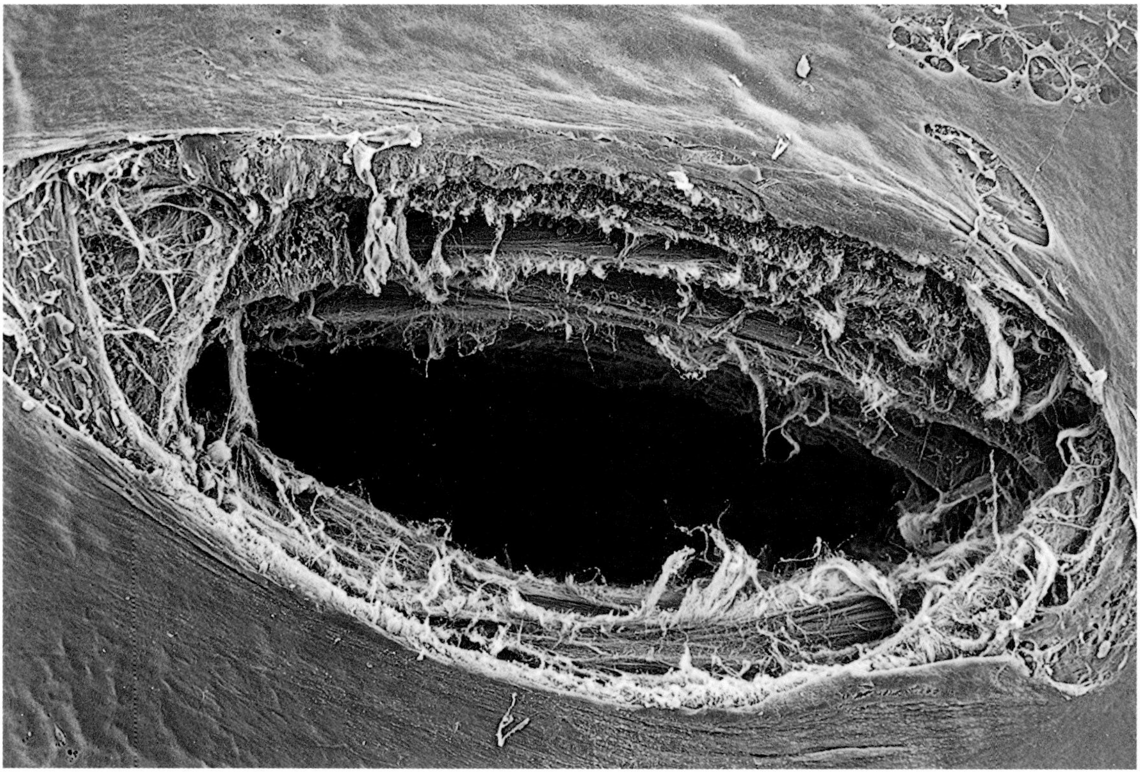

Because the shape of the needle tip is believed to be important to CSF leak,[7-8] several different types are available (Fig. 4.5). While there are minor differences in the resulting leakage of CSF due to different needle points, the main difference relates to the OD of the needle. However, even the smallest (29 gauge) needles can create holes through which CSF can leak, and headaches cannot be totally eliminated.

Combined spinal/epidural needles are also available (Fig. 4.6). The method (see p. 124) involves inserting a Tuohy needle into the epidural space, following which a 26 or 29 gauge needle is passed through it into the subarachnoid space.

Fig. 4.5. Spinal needle tips.

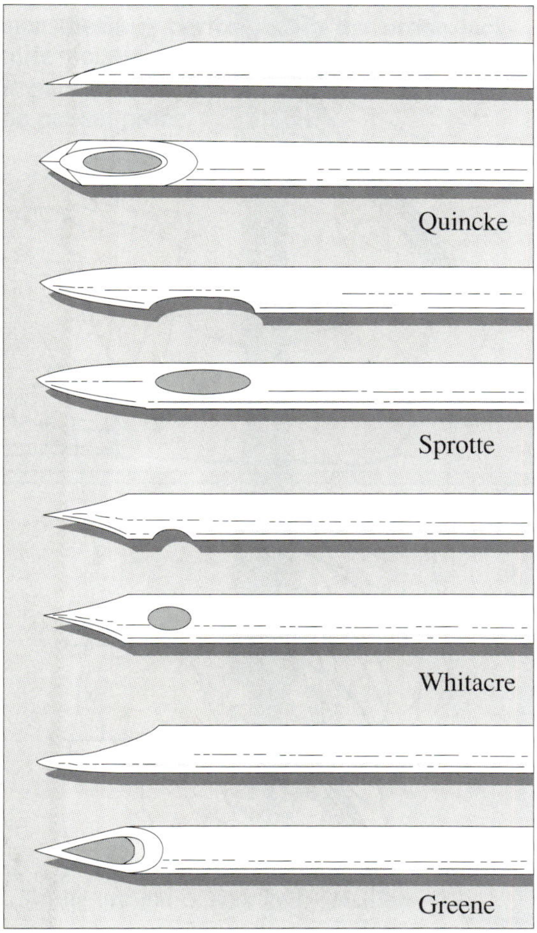

Fig. 4.6. Combined spinal/epidural needle (B. Braun)

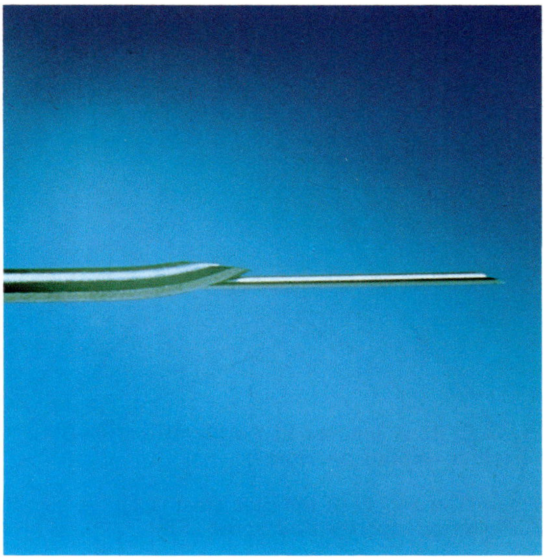

Midline approach

Having chosen the appropriate intervertebral space, the skin over one of the adjacent vertebral spines is held firmly by the second and third fingers of the non-dominant hand. This stops the skin from moving as the needle is inserted through it (Fig. 4.9).

The needle is directed slightly cephalad and equidistant between the two lumbar spines. The bevel should be aligned so as to separate the longitudinal fibres of the dura rather than cut them (Fig. 4.10).

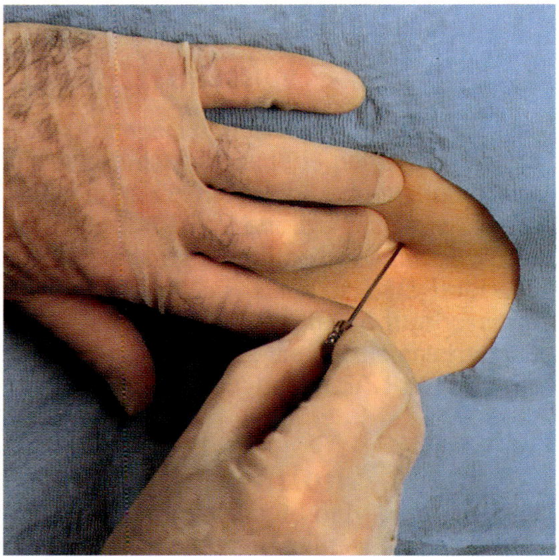

Fig. 4.9.

Fig. 4.10. The effect that the direction of the needle bevel has on the hole left in the dura mater. If the bevel is oriented so that it cuts across the longitudinal dural fibres (right), the fibres of the dura mater are cut and a hole is left. If the bevel space separates the fibres (left), there is less damage and the resulting hole is much smaller.

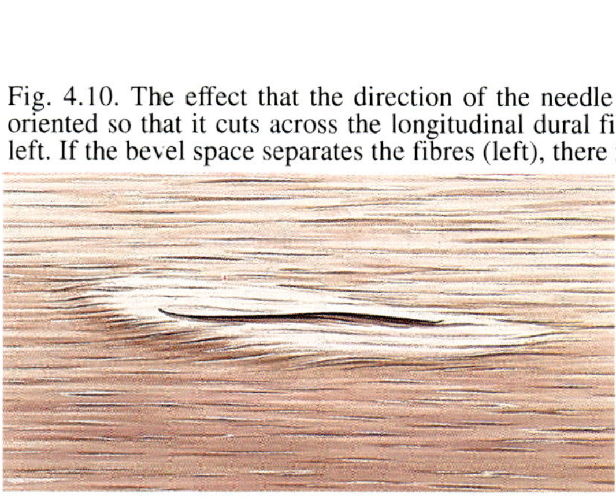

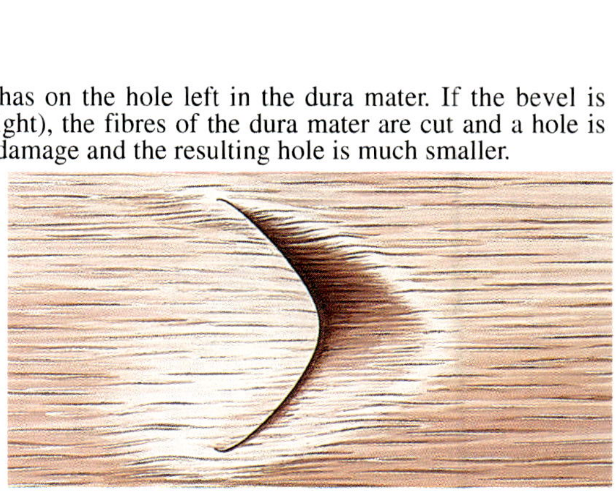

On advancing the needle, the various ligaments are identified by their "feel", the interspinous ligament being firmer than the subcutaneous tissue and the ligamentum flavum being even more firm. The needle is advanced approximately 1 cm past the ligamentum flavum. Sometimes there is a distinct click as the dura is punctured (Fig. 4.11).

The stylet is removed and the needle hub examined for CSF (Fig. 4.12). If none appears after a reasonable time, the needle is advanced another 0.5 cm.

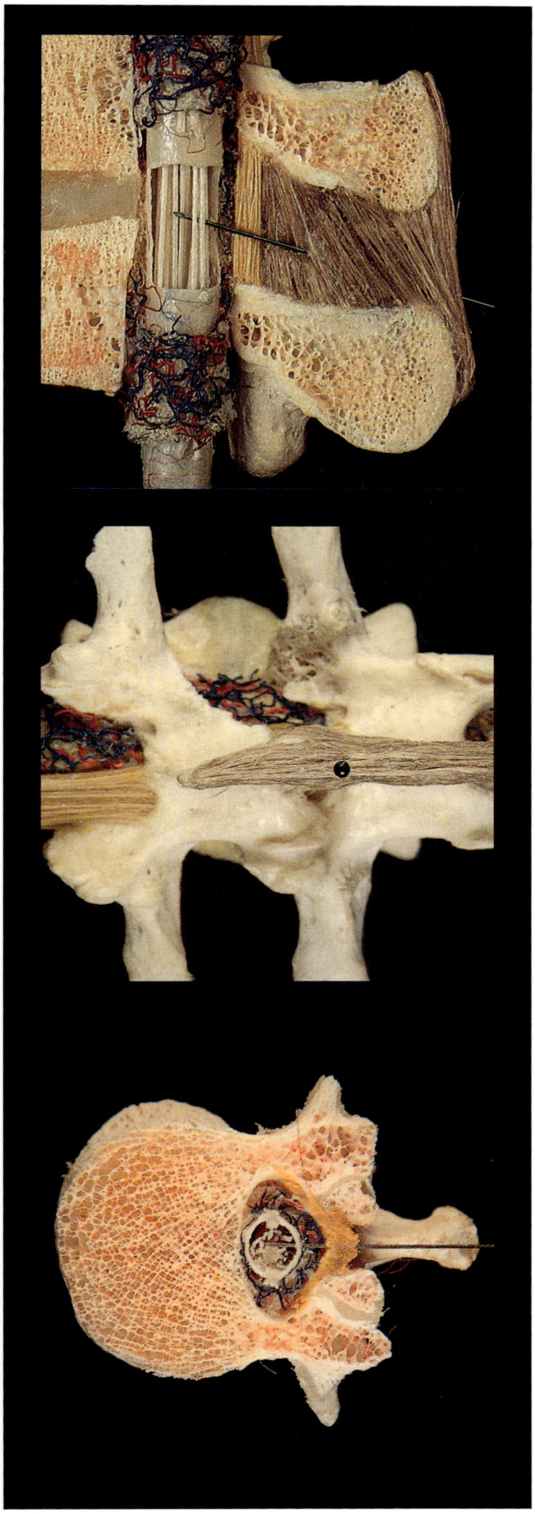

Fig. 4.11. Needle directions.
Anatomical models Erling Worm Skole, M.D.

Fig. 4.12. The needle hub is examined for CSF.

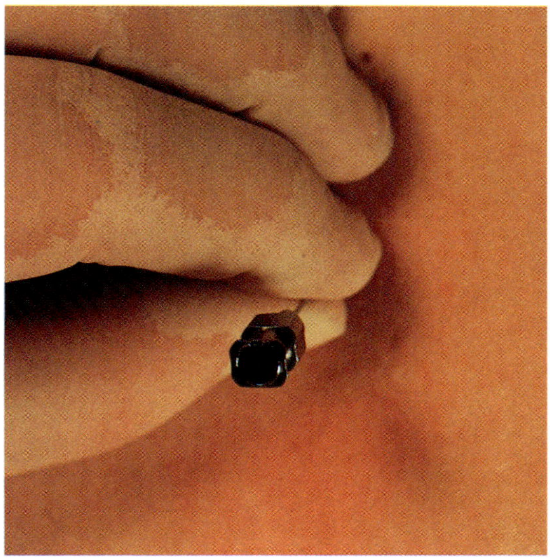

Should bone be contacted within 2-3 cm of the skin, it is probably the lamina of the lower vertebra (Fig. 4.13) and the needle must be redirected more cephalad. To do this with a thin spinal needle requires withdrawing it back to the subcutaneous tissue before re-aligning and re-advancing.

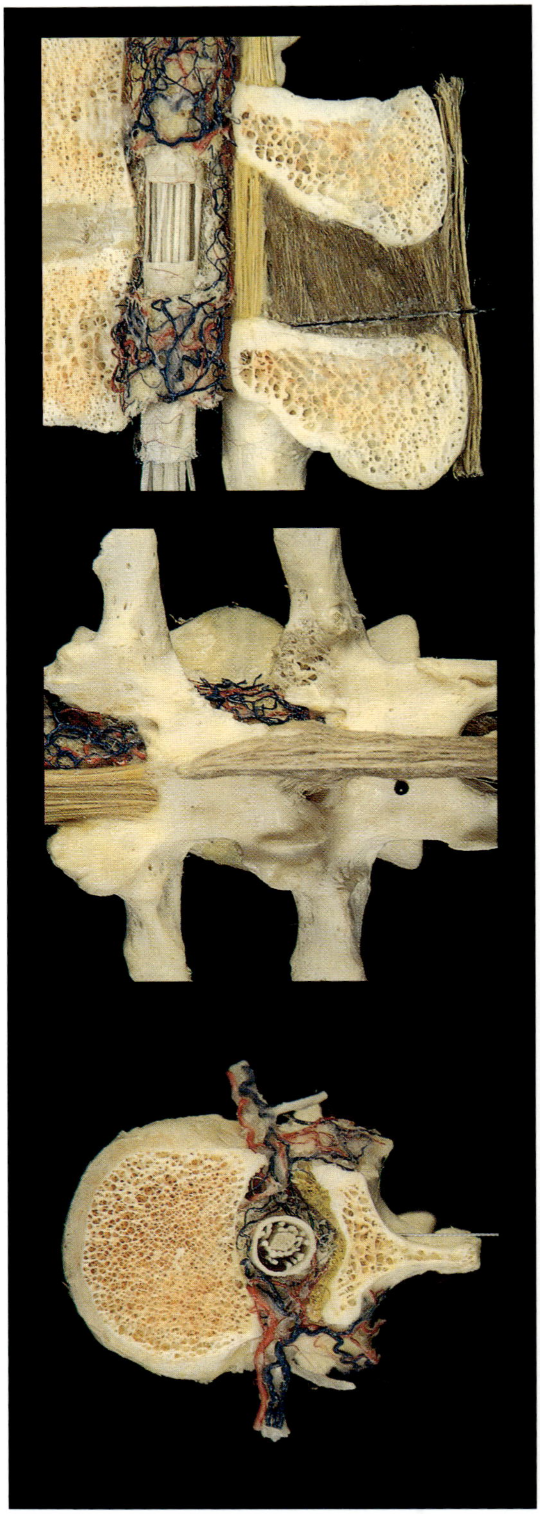

Fig. 4.13.Needle directions.
Anatomical models Erling Worm Skole, M.D.

If the initial insertion is too cephalad, the spinous process above may be contacted and a more caudad approach is required (Fig. 4.14).

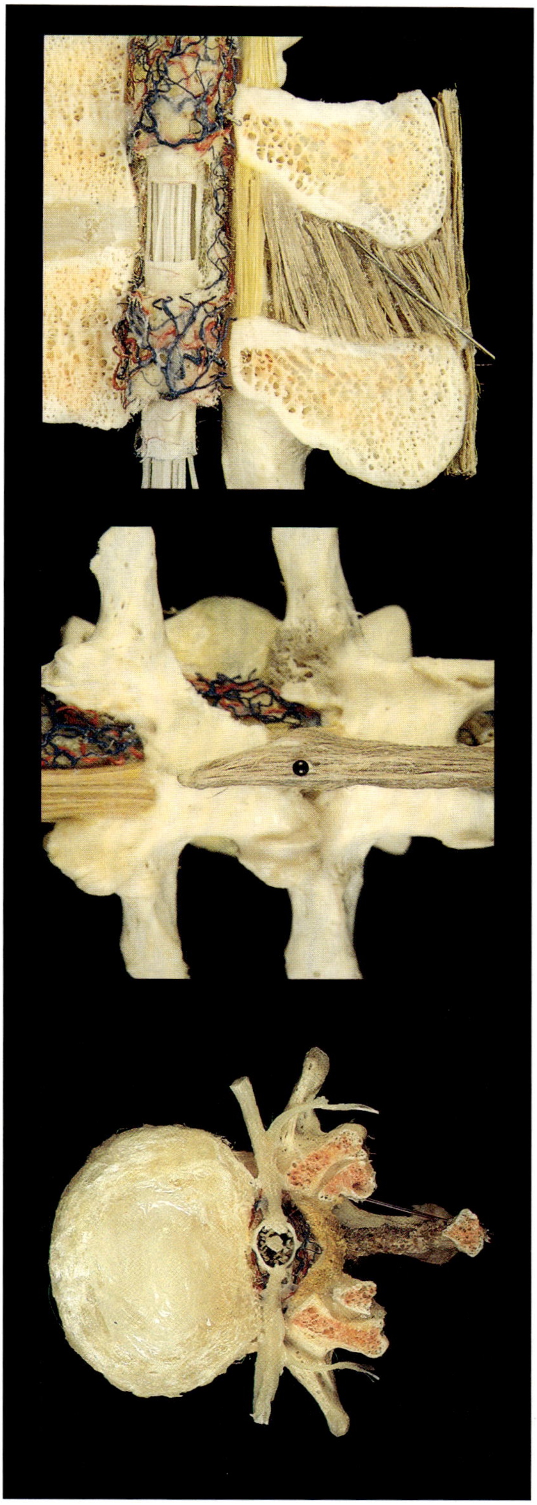

Fig. 4.14. Needle directions.
Anatomical models Erling Worm Skole, M.D.

If bone is felt deep in the back it is probably the anterior wall of the spinal canal (Fig. 4.15). In this case, the stylet is removed and the needle withdrawn slowly while the hub is examined for CSF.

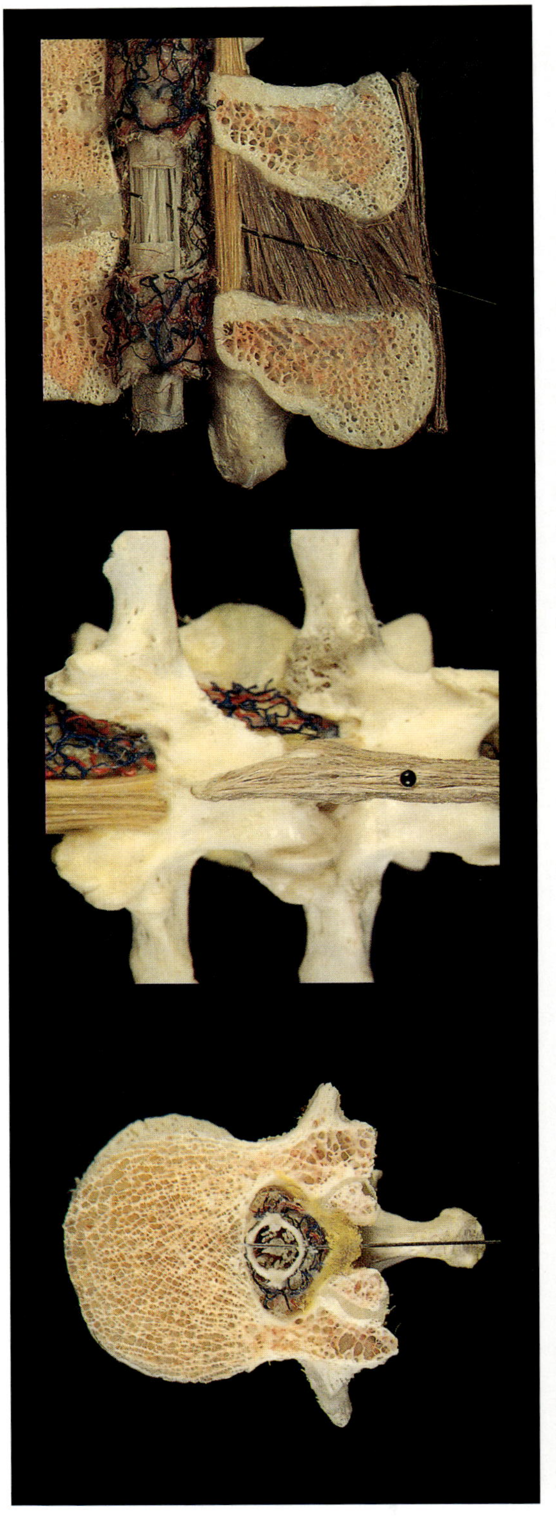

Fig. 4.15. Needle directions.
Anatomical models Erling Worm Skole, M.D.

An introducer is usually employed for needles of 25 gauge or finer. This is inserted until it is in the ligamentum flavum. The spinal needle is now passed through it into the subarachnoid space (Fig. 4.16).

If bone is contacted before reaching the spinal canal this indicates that the introducer is not properly inserted. The needle should be withdrawn into the introducer, which is itself then withdrawn and redirected, usually more cephalad.

If no CSF is seen in the needle hub the following possibilities should be considered:

1. Not enough time has elapsed for the fluid to appear. With a 29 gauge needle and using the lateral position, this may take 60-70 sec. Although aspiration is often recommended, its value is questionable. However, the rapid withdrawel of the stylet can act as an aspiration leaving a drop of CSF in the clear plastic hub.

2. The needle bevel is not completely in the subarachnoid space. Try advancing the needle an additional 1-2 mm and rotating it through 90^{0} to 180^{0}.

3. The needle is not in the subarachnoid space, and must be re-inserted. Before doing this, withdraw the needle slowly as the tip may have gone beyond the subarachnoid space anteriorly (Fig. 4.15).

Do not inject local anaesthetic until CSF is clearly identified and a free flow obtained.

In difficult cases, decide sooner, rather than later, either to seek more experienced help or to abandon the technique. Frequent repeated needling is to be avoided. Apart from discomfort, it may cause multiple dural puncture holes, and possible neural damage.

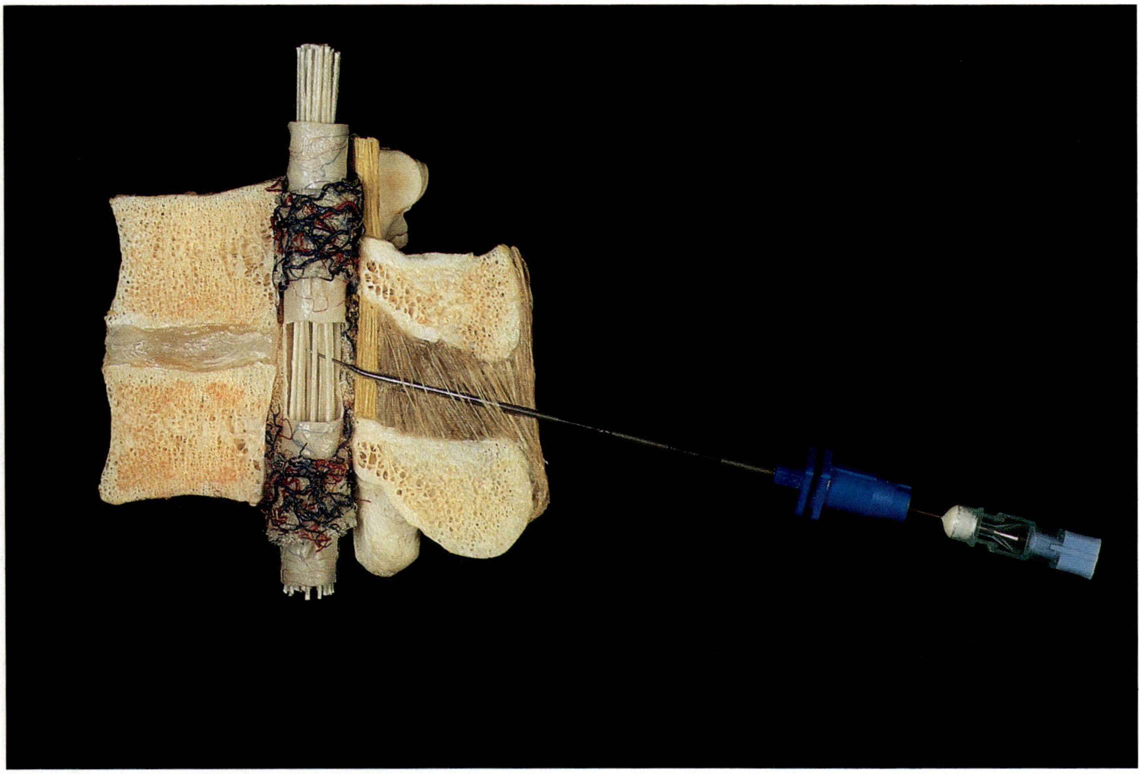

Fig. 4.16. Spinal needle passed through an epidural needle. Anatomical models Erling Worm Skole,

Continuous spinal anaesthesia

Continuous spinal anaesthesia (CSA) was introduced by Dean in 1907, who left the spinal needle in place during the operation.[13] In 1940, Lemmon introduced the malleable needle and split mattress technique to overcome the problems of needle trauma and needle breakage.[14,15] Tuohy (1944) employed a no. 4 ureteral catheter inserted through a 15 gauge needle into the subarachnoid space.[16] Since that time, the diameter of the needles and catheters employed for continuous spinal anaesthesia have decreased. Seventeen and 18 gauge epidural needles have been used to introduce 19 and 20 gauge epidural catheters. Although continuous spinal anaesthesia has advantages, it has not achieved the popularity of continuous epidural blockade due to the perceived high incidence of postdural puncture headache (vide infra).[17,18]

Advantages and disadvantages[18-21]

Continuous spinal anaesthesia has advantages over both single-dose spinal and continuous epidural blockade:

1. The onset of anaesthesia is rapid.

2. Spinal anaesthesia requires 10-15 times less local anaesthetic than is needed for epidural blockade, thus eliminating the possibility of systemic toxic reactions and total spinal anaesthesia.

3. It may be instituted after patient positioning, minimizing the potential for cardiovascular instability.

4. Careful titration of sensory blockade decreases the likelihood of cardiovascular instability during induction.

5. By employing low doses of short-acting local anaesthetics (procaine or lidocaine) the recovery period is shortened.

6. The duration of analgesia can be prolonged indefinitely.

7. Subarachnoid narcotics may be administered at the end of the surgical procedure to provide long-lasting postoperative analgesia.

A disadvantage of CSA is the additional time required to insert the catheter, which occasionally is difficult or impossible. Nevertheless, CSA is particularly useful in the following situations:

1. In critically ill patients where slow incremental dosing minimizes haemodynamic changes,

2. Whenever the duration of the operation may exceed the duration of the single-dose technique,

3. For short operations when intermittent injections of small doses of short-acting local anaesthestics can be given to facilitate rapid recovery.

Catheters for continuous spinal anaesthesia

Until recently, the majority of continuous spinal anaesthetics were performed with commercially available epidural catheters inserted through a 17 or 18G epidural needle. A 24G catheter, which can be inserted through a 20G needle is also available (Fig. 4.21). Several smaller gauge catheters, designed to decrease the incidence of post-dural puncture headache, have been introduced in the USA, including a 27G polyurethane catheter (Preferred Medical), a 28G nylon catheter (Kendall Healthcare) and a 28 and 32G polyimide catheter (Rüsch).[21-23] The 27 and 28G catheters are compatible with most 22G spinal needles and the 32G catheter can be inserted through most 25 or 26G needles.

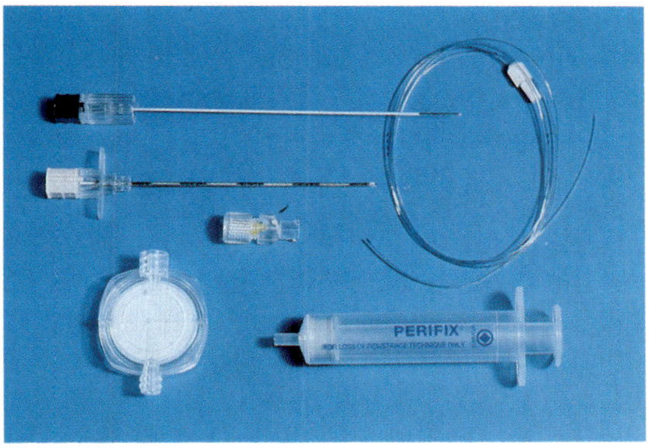

Fig. 4.21. Spinal set with 20G needle and 24G catheter (B. Braun).

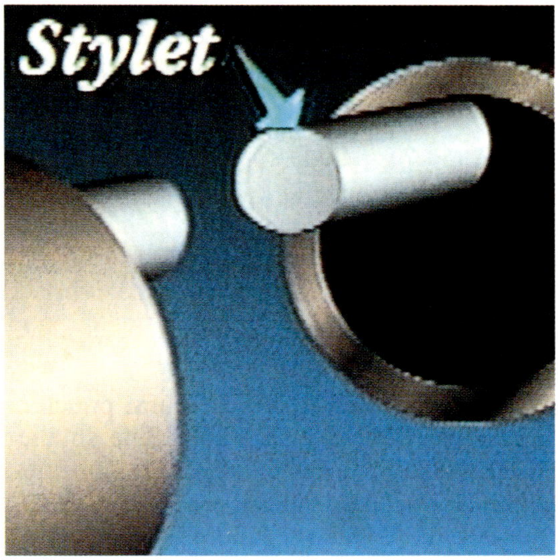

Fig. 4.22. Cutaway section of 32G catheter showing integrated stylet.

The different catheters have their own advantages and disadvantages. Those with an integral stylet are stiffer and are sometimes more difficult to insert. However, they have a relatively high tensile strength. The polyurethane and nylon catheters are softer and thread more easily, but have lower tensile strength (Table 4.2).

Microcatheter development

The 32 gauge polyimide catheter was chosen for its physical characteristics and its lack of biological reactivity. Initial studies were promising, but also troublesome.[21] Lack of tensile strength and kinking were major problems. A 0.0076 mm stainless steel stylet was initially employed in the conventional manner, being withdrawn after catheter placement. However, leaving the stylet in place (and later bonding it to the polyimide) greatly improved tensile strength and eliminated the problem of kinking (Fig. 4.22). The stylet also made the catheter radio-opaque.

Table 4.2. Commercially available catheters.

Manufacturer	Catheter material	Gauge	Compatible needle gauge	Break strength (lbs)	Elongation* (%)
Rüsch	Teflon	20**	18	3.0	280
Rüsch	Nylon	20**	18	3.9	290
Rüsch	Polyimide	32	25 or 26	2.5	100***
Rüsch	Polyimide	28	22	7.4	100***
Kendall	Nylon	28	22	1.25	550
Pref.Med.	Polyurethane	27	22	1.30	475

* Elongation of 1" length of catheter prior to breaking
** Epidural catheter
*** Stylet elongates 1%, polyimide elongates 100%

Combined spinal and epidural anaesthesia

In recent years there has been interest in combining spinal with continuous epidural blockade to obtain both a rapid onset and a prolonged duration of anaesthesia.[24-26] The usual indication for this is urgent Caesarean section, although any procedure where postoperative epidural analgesia is used is also an indication. The patient can be made ready for surgery quickly, and the nerve block maintained and continued into the postoperative period using an epidural catheter.

The principle is to locate the epidural space with an epidural needle, through which a spinal needle is advanced into the subarachnoid space (Fig. 4.25).

Because the spinal needle is held in place only by the dura mater, it is possible for it to be displaced when connecting the syringe to it or while injecting the local anaesthetic. This is a critical point in the combined spinal-epidural method and care must be taken to ensure that the spinal needle is not dislodged during these manipulations. Once the tip of the spinal needle is properly positioned in the CSF, the usual dose of local anaesthetic can be injected. This produces rapid onset of profound anaesthesia but increases the risk of hypotension. The spinal needle is withdrawn and an epidural catheter passed into the epidural space (Fig. 4.26). Local anaesthetic is not injected through the epidural catheter, if the spinal block is sufficient for the operation. However, should the spinal be inadequate or the operation exceed its duration, general anaesthesia can be avoided by using the epidural catheter to extend the block. Alternatively, a two-stage technique can be used, where half the usual spinal dose is given and the block extended later with incremental epidural injections, the objective being to reduce the incidence and severity of hypotension, particularly in pregnant or debilitated patients. Theoretically, sympathectic block will be less with the two stage technique because the spinal block should be low. This, combined with a slower onset of epidural blockade, allows more time for compensatory vasoconstriction to occur, reducing the likelihood of hypotension. Regardless of whether a one- or two-stage technique is used, the epidural catheter can be used for prolonged, postoperative analgesia.

Fig. 4.25. A spinal needle is passed through the epidural needle to enter the subarachnoid space. Anatomical model ErlingWorm Skole, M.D.

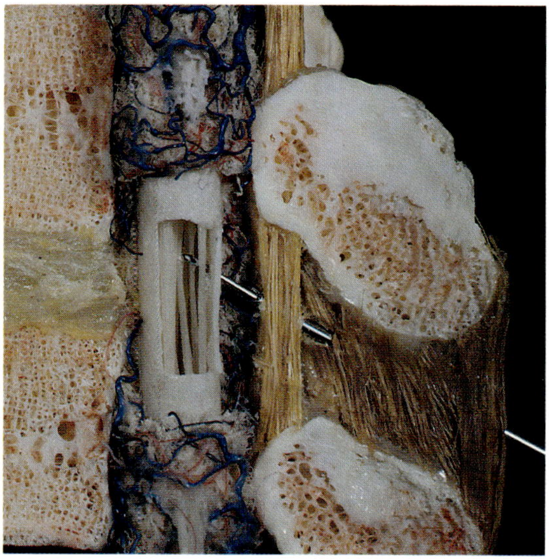

Fig. 4.26. After removing the spinal needle a catheter is threaded into the epidural space. Anatomical model Erling Worm Skole, M.D.

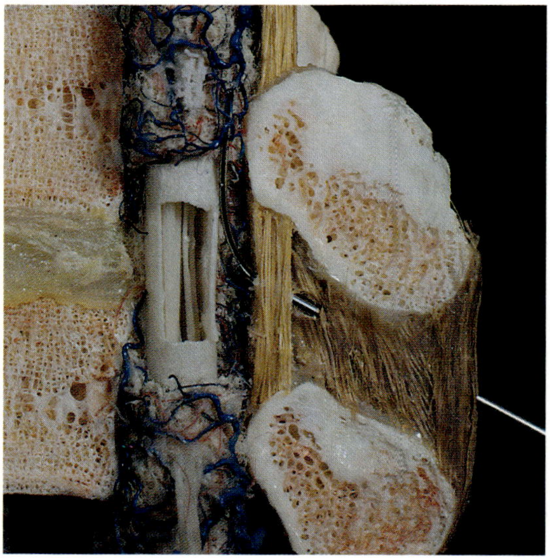

Technique

The epidural needle is inserted into the ligamentum flavum at L2-3 or L3-4 using either the midline or paramedian approach. The stylet is removed and the needle advanced into the epidural space using a loss of resistance technique (Fig. 4.25). The needle hub is examined for leakage of CSF or blood. If neither appears, the spinal needle is inserted along the epidural needle and pushed forward to puncture the dura mater. The stylet of the spinal needle is removed and CSF should appear at the hub.

A suitable dose of local anaesthetic is now injected through the spinal needle, which is then withdrawn completely. An epidural catheter is now advanced along the epidural needle so that 3-5 cm lies within the epidural space (Fig. 4.26). The catheter, being much larger than the spinal needle, cannot gain access to the subarachnoid space through the hole made by the spinal needle. The epidural needle is now withdrawn over the catheter, which is taped securely to the patient´s back.

Spinal anaesthesia will develop within a few minutes and provided the height of the block is adequate, the operation may begin. If the height of block is too low then 5 mL aliquots of local anaesthetic suitable for epidural blockade (e.g. 2% lidocaine or 0.5% bupivacaine) are injected down the catheter every 5 min until the anaesthesia is satisfactory.

In most cases the spinal blockade will be adequate and epidural injections are not required until the anaesthesia is due to wear off. However, the spinal anaesthesia may be reinforced by an epidural injection of an opioid, e.g. 3-5 mg of morphine or 25-50 μg of fentanyl. Alternatively, a continuous infusion of a local anaesthetic/opioid mixture may be started, e.g. 5 $mL{\cdot}h^{-1}$ of 0.25% bupivacaine containing morphine 0.25 mg (0.05 $mg{\cdot}mL^{-1}$) or fentanyl 25 μg (5 $\mu g{\cdot}mL^{-1}$). By the time the spinal anaesthesia wears off, the epidural infusion will be exerting an analgesic effect.

References

1. Messahel FM, Robinson JS, Mathews ET (1983) Factors affecting cerebrospinal fluid flow in two spinal needles. Br J Anaesth 55: 169

2. Gerrish SP, Peacook JE (1987) Variations in the flow of cerebrospinal fluid through spinal needles. Br J Anaesth 59:1465

3. Eldor J (1990) A device for small-bore spinal needles for immediate detection of CSF. Can J Anaesth 37:145

4. Dittmann M, Schäfer HG, Ulrich J, Bond-Taylor W (1988) Anatomical re-evaluation of lumbar dura mater with regard to postspinal headache. Effect of dural puncture. Anaesthesia 43:635

5. Fink BR, Walker S (1989) Orientation of fibers in human dorsal lumbar dura mater in relation to lumbar puncture. Anesth Analg 69:768

6. Mihic DN (1986) Postspinal headaches, needle surfaces and longitudinal orientation of the dural fibers. Results of a survey. Reg Anaesth 9:54

7. Janes EF, Pennefather S, Wilkinsonn K (1989) Fluid flow through dural puncture sites. Anaesthesia 44:1011

8. Cruickshank RH, Hopkinson JM (1989). Fluid flow through dural puncture sites. An in vitro comparison of needle point types. Anaesthesia 44:415

9. Ready LB, Woodland RV, Haschke RH (1985) Spinal needle angle affects rate of fluid leak across human dura. Anesthesiology 65:A241

10. Ready LB, Cuplin S, Haeschke RH, Nessly M (1989) Spinal needle determinants of rate of transdural fluid leak. Anesth Analg 69:457

11. Hatfalvi BI (1977) The dynamics of post-spinal headache. Headache 17:64-66

12. Taylor JA (1940) Lumbosacral subarachnoid tap. J Urol 43:561

13. Dean HP (1907) Discussion on the relative value of inhalation and injection methods of inducing anaesthesia. Br Med J 5:869

14. Lemmon WT (1940) A method for continuous spinal anesthesia. Ann Surg 111: 141

15. Lemmon WT, Paschal GW (1941) Continuous spinal anesthesia: with observations on the first 500 cases. Pennsylvania Medical Journal 44:975

16. Tuohy EB (1944) Continuous spinal anesthesia: its usefulness and technique involved. Anesthesia 5: 142

17. Denny N, Masters R, Pearson D, et al. (1987) Postdural puncture headache after continuous spinal anesthesia. Anesth Analg 66: 791

18. Hurley RJ (1989) Continuous spinal anesthesia. Int Anesth Clin. 27:46

19. Giuffrida JG, Bizzari DV, Masi R, et al. (1972) Continuous procaine spinal anesthesia for cesarean section. Anesth Analg 51:117

20. Bizzari D, Giuffrida JG, Brandoc L, Fierro FE (1964) Continuous spinal anesthesia using a special needle and catheter. Anest Analg 43:393

21. Hurley RJ, Lambert DH (1990) Continuous spinal anesthesia with a microcatheter technique: preliminary experience. Anesth Analg 70:97

22. Hurley RJ, Lambert DH (1990) Microcatheters for continuous spinal anesthesia (letter to the editor). Anesth Analg 71:201

23. Wissler RN, Bjoraker DG (1990) Continuous spinal anesthesia microcatheters. Anesthesiol Rev 17:49

24. Brownridge P (1981) Epidural and subarachnoid analgesia for elective Caesarean section. Anaesthesia 36:70

25. Rawal N, Schollin J, Wesström G (1988) Epidural versus combined spinal epidural block for cesarean section. Acta Anaesthesiol Scand 32:61

26. Carrie LES (1990) Extradural, spinal or combined block for obstetric surgical anaesthesia. Brit J Anaesth 65:225

Chapter 5

Clinical considerations

Clinical rationale for spinal anaesthesia

Scientific studies indicate that in specific clinical situations, spinal anaesthesia has significant advantages over other anaesthetic methods.

Many other studies indicate an advantage for epidural blockade over general anaesthesia, particularly when the epidural is continued for 24 h, or more, postoperatively. Similar results might be expected with continuous spinal anaesthesia, but there are no good data yet published.

Surgical stress response

Trauma, including surgery, activates nociceptive impulses that are transmitted to the brain. These, in turn, activate efferent impulses to certain endocrine organs, causing endocrine and metabolic alterations which occur soon after the start of surgery and continue into the postoperative period. Operations performed with general inhalation anaesthesia increase plasma concentrations of cortisol, aldosterone, renin, vasopressin, growth hormone, epinephrine, norepinephrine, dextrose and lactate[1]. These changes are related to surgical trauma, and inhalation anaesthesia does not inhibit the afferent and efferent pathways responsible for this so-called stress response.[2-4]

Spinal anaesthesia itself does not alter endocrine function or metabolic activity prior to the start of surgery, except for modest increases in blood glucose and decreases in catecholamine levels.[3,4] The changes in plasma catecholamine levels relate to the level of block.[4] Spinal anaesthesia to the upper thoracic dermatomal level results in a decrease in arterial epinephrine and norepinephrine concentrations while low thoracic blocks cause no significant changes.

Although general anaesthesia does not markedly influence the stress response to surgery, spinal anaesthesia extending to the mid-thoracic dermatomal level prevents significant change in either epinephrine or norepinephrine levels intraoperatively or postoperatively. With regard to metabolic alterations, spinal anaesthesia inhibits the surgically induced increase in blood glucose and cortisol levels[3,5] (Table 5.1).

The blockade of either nociceptive afferent or efferent pathways, or both, is believed to be responsible for the inhibition of the endocrine and metabolic changes due to surgical stress. The inhibition of the release of pituitary hormones by spinal anaesthesia probably relates to the blockade of afferent nociceptive pathways. However, the absence of increased cortisol secretion during operations performed under spinal anaesthesia may be due to inhibition of either efferent or, more likely, afferent fibres, which in turn prevents the

Table 5.1. Effect of spinal anaesthesia on surgically induced changes in endocrine/metabolic functions.

Endocrine/metabolic parameter	Surgery	Spinal anaesthesia
Norepinephrine *	Increased	Inhibited
Epinephrine *	Increased	Inhibited
Glucose	Increased	Inhibited
Free fatty acids *	Increased	Inhibited
Insulin	Unchanged	Unchanged
Growth hormone	Increased	Inhibited
Cortisol	Increased	Inhibited

* Depends on level of anaesthesia

Table 5.2. Intraoperative blood loss during general and spinal anaesthesia. Reproduced with permission from Covino[16]

Author	Surgical procedure	Average blood loss (mL) General anaesthesia	Spinal anaesthesia	Difference (mL)
Aitkenhead et al [6], 1978	Large bowel surgery	430 ±109	27 ± 4	403
Thorburn et al [7], 1980	Total hip arthroplasty	848 ± 61	420 ± 41	428
McKenzie et al [8], 1980	Femoral neck fracture	264 ± 46	261 ± 47	3
McKenzie et al [9], 1984	Femoral neck fracture	261 ± 37	278 ± 36	-17
Hedenstierna et al[10], 1985	Total hip arthroplasty	1,850	850	1,000
McKenzie et al [11], 1985	Femoral neck fracture	243 ± 47	348 ± 64	-105
Cook et al [12], 1986	Vascular surgery	792 ± 440	560 ± 340	232
Johnson et al [13], 1986	Major hip surgery	1,299 ± 678	1,264 ± 697	35
Svartling et al [2], 1986	Femoral neck fracture	583 ± 72	377 ± 43	206
Valentin et al [14], 1986	Femoral neck fracture	-----------------------(Significantly less)---------------		
Davis et al [15], 1987	Total hip arthroplasty	671 ± 335	527 ± 232	144

release of ACTH from the pituitary gland. Similarly, the lower levels of epinephrine and norepinephrine during operations with high thoracic spinal anaesthesia probably relate to the blockade of efferent autonomic pathways to the adrenal medulla.

Blood loss

A number of investigators have evaluated the influence of anaesthesia on perioperative blood loss during various surgical procedures, such as total hip replacements and prostatectomies.[2,6-15] (Table 5.2). For example, Thorburn and co-workers[7] reported an average perioperative blood loss of 420 ± 41 mL during total hip replacements performed under spinal anaesthesia compared to 848± 61 mL with general anaesthesia. Davis and colleagues[15] reported an average blood loss of 527 mL when total hip replacements were performed under spinal anaesthesia compared to 671 mL with general anaesthesia.

The decrease in blood loss during spinal anaesthesia is believed to be due to the hypotension produced by the sympathetic block. Hypotensive anaesthesia with halothane and nitroprusside also results in similar reductions in intraoperative blood loss.

The decreased blood loss during certain surgical procedures performed with spinal anaesthesia results in a decreased requirement for blood transfusion (Table 5.3). This is particularly important because of the concern regarding the possibility of transmitting AIDS and hepatitis via blood transfusions. Fewer blood transfusions were necessary in patients undergoing total hip replacement[3,7,15], transurethral prostactectomy[17] or large bowel surgery[6] with spinal anaesthesia compared to general anaesthesia.

Table 5.3. Frequency of blood transfusion during general and spinal anaesthesia. Reproduced with permission from Covino[16]

Author	Surgical procedure	Number of transfusions General Anaesthesia	Spinal Anaesthesia
Aitkenhead et al [6], 1978	Large bowel surgery	8 (30%)	0
Thorburn et al [7], 1980	Total hip arthroplasty	33 (70%)	4 (10%)
McGowan and Smith [17], 1980	Transurethral prostate resection	17 (34%)	16 (32%)
Davis et al [3], 1987	Total hip arthroplasty	12 (24%)	4 (8%)
Davis et al [15], 1987	Total hip arthroplasty	11 (57%)	4 (17%)

Thromboembolism

The incidence of deep venous thrombosis in patients having elective hip replacements is reported to be 54% with general anaesthesia compared to 29% with spinal anaesthesia.[7] Evidence of deep venous thrombosis was present in 76.2% of elderly patients in whom repair of fractured neck of the femur was performed under general anaesthesia and 40% with spinal anaesthesia.[11] These results are attributed to an increase in blood flow to the lower extremities as a result of the sympathetic blockade that accompanies spinal or epidural anaesthesia.[18,19]

Pulmonary complications

Conflicting results have been reported concerning the postoperative pulmonary status of patients given either spinal or general anaesthesia for various surgical procedures. A significant decrease in PaO_2 occurred 1 h following repair of fractured neck of the femur performed under general anaesthesia.[8] No significant change occurred when spinal anaesthesia was used. On the other hand, a significantly lower PaO_2 and higher $PaCO_2$ occurred 4 h following total knee or hip arthroplasty performed under spinal anaesthesia compared to patients given general anaesthesia.[10] The incidence of postoperative respiratory infections was 33% in patients given general anaesthesia for lower limb vascular surgery, but only 16% with spinal anaesthesia.[12] However, in another study, 35% of patients developed postoperative respiratory infections when spinal anaesthesia was used for repair of fractured neck of the femur compared to 24% in patients who received general anaesthesia.[20] In this study, the patients given spinal anaesthesia had a higher incidence of preoperative respiratory problems and this may have influenced the incidence of postoperative respiratory complications.

Miscellaneous complications

In a retrospective study, 23.1% of patients having colonic or rectal anastomoses with general anaesthesia suffered anastomotic dehiscence postoperatively, compared to 7.4% of patients who received spinal anaesthesia.[6] A significant relationship also exists between the incidence of postoperative hip dislocation following major hip surgery and the anaesthetic technique.[10] No hip dislocations occurred in 112 patients having spinal anaesthesia whereas 6 of 132 patients suffered hip dislocations postoperatively when general anaesthesia was used. Because of this difference in the incidence of postoperative hip dislocations, the average postoperative stay in this particular study was 3.5 days shorter in the patients given spinal anaesthesia. Other studies fail to indicate any significant difference in duration of hospitalization as a function of the anaesthetic utilized for specific surgical procedures.[13]

Mortality studies

Several studies compared the incidence of short-term and long-term mortality in patients given spinal or general anaesthesia (Table 5.4). The majority of these involve geriatric

Table 5.4 Postoperative mortality following major lower limb orthopaedic procedures performed with spinal or general anaesthesia. Reproduced with permission from Covino[16]

	Cumulative mortality (%)									
	2 weeks		4 weeks		6 months		12 months		24 months	
Author	GA	Spinal	GA	Spinal	GA	Spinal	GA	Spinal	GA	Spinal
McLaren et al[20], 1978	24	0	31	4	-	-	-	-	-	-
McKenzie et al[8], 1980	12	4	16	10	-	-	-	-	-	-
Davis et al[21], 1981	-	-	13	5	-	-	-	-	-	-
McKenzie et al[9], 1984	16	4	17	11	-	-	33	36	-	-
Valentin et al[14], 1986	6	3	8	6	14	14	20	20	28	31

patients having lower limb orthopaedic procedures. For example, in one study involving 55 patients, average age 76 years, 31% given a general anaesthesia died during a 1 month postoperative observation period.[20] On the other hand, only one death (4%) occurred in patients who received spinal anaesthesia. A second study found a 16% mortality rate within 2 weeks following repair of fractured neck of the femur performed with general anaesthesia compared to a mortality rate of only 4% with spinal anaesthesia.[9] However, long-term survival rates did not differ. For example, although a significantly lower mortality rate was observed during the 2 week postoperative period when spinal anaesthesia was employed, the survival rates between 2 months and 1 year were equivalent.[9] A large study of 578 patients followed for 2 years after surgical repair of femoral neck fractures performed with either spinal or general anaesthesia, detected a slight but not significantly lower mortality rate in the spinal anaesthesia group during the 2 to 4 week postoperative period.[14] However, survival rates were nearly identical at 6 to 24 months following surgery in both groups. It is interesting that in these mortality studies many of the deaths that occurred during the first month after operation in the general anaesthetic population were related to thromboembolic complications. On the other hand, relatively few deaths were attributed to thromboembolic complications in patients who received spinal anaesthesia. These data again suggest that spinal anaesthesia results in a lower incidence of deep venous thrombosis.

Comparison of spinal and epidural anaesthesia

Spinal and epidural anaesthesia are both effective in preventing pain in surgical and obstetrical patients. The primary advantage of epidural anaesthesia relates to placing a catheter in the epidural space and providing continuous analgesia for long periods of time. It is also possible to place a catheter in the subarachnoid space and provide continuous spinal analgesia. However, this technique has not been popular until now because of the high incidence of post-dural puncture headache (see p 122). Both techniques have advantages.

Epidural anaesthesia is advantageous since:

1. It does not involve puncture of the dura and thus is not associated with post-dural puncture headache. However, accidental dural puncture during the performance of epidural anaesthesia occurs in 0.5-1% of patients.

2. The slower onset of sympathetic blockade results in less hypotension.

3. A discrete band of analgesia can be produced by thoracic epidural blockade.

4. Separation of sensory and motor fibre blockade is possible with low concentrations of bupivacaine.

Spinal anaesthesia also has many advantages:

1. It is relatively easy to perform.

2. The endpoint of proper location of the needle tip is more objective due to the presence of CSF in the needle.

3. The onset of anaesthesia is more rapid.

4. The anaesthesia is more profound.

5. The level of anaesthesia can be controlled by the use of anaesthetic solutions of varying baricity and patient position.

6. Local anaesthetic induced systemic toxicity should never occur even if an accidental intravascular injection is made.

The major disadvantages of spinal anaesthesia relative to epidural anaesthesia are the ever present possibility of post-dural puncture headache and the hypotension which may occur owing to rapid blockade of sympathetic fibres. Also, the chance of neural damage may be greater if an irritating substance is accidentally injected intrathecally. Access to the subarachnoid space is limited to the lumbar region, while epidural block can be performed at any lumbar, thoracic or cervical intervertebral space.

The cardiovascular effects of spinal and epidural anaesthesia were compared in volunteers who received either hyperbaric 5% lidocaine intrathecally or 2% lidocaine epidurally sufficient to produce an average T5 level of sensory analgesia[22] (Table 5.5). Arterial pressure fell by 21% in the spinal group compared to an average decrease of only 9% following epidural blockade. Cardiac output decreased approximately 18% in the spinal group compared to 5% in the epidural group. Stroke volume decreased 25% following induction of spinal anaesthesia, compared to 10% with epidural anaesthesia. The increase in heart rate and decrease in peripheral resistance were similar in both groups. The differential haemodynamic effects are no doubt due to the slower onset of sympathetic blockade following administration of local anaesthetics into the epidural space, which allows time for compensatory cardiovascular changes. The degree and extent of sympathetic blockade following spinal anaesthesia may also be greater than that which occurs following epidural blockade. When epinephrine (5 $\mu g \cdot mL^{-1}$) was added to the epidural local anaesthetic solution, peripheral resistance and mean blood pressure decreased while pulse rate, cardiac output and stroke volume increased. These beta effects of epinephrine are due to its systemic absorption.

Both spinal and epidural anaesthesia can produce effective surgical anaesthesia provided the techniques are properly performed and appropriate anaesthetic solutions employed. A comparison in orthopaedic patients who received either 15 mg of hyperbaric bupivacaine intrathecally or 100 mg of bupivacaine epidurally revealed that spinal anaesthesia produced more satisfactory anaesthesia.[23] Although a T5 pin prick level of analgesia was achieved in both groups, supplemental parenteral analgesia or sedation was required in 73% of the epidural patients compared to only 6% of the spinal patients. In addition, the incidence of tourniquet pain was significantly greater with epidural anaesthesia.

In summary, both spinal and epidural anaesthesia are effective for surgical and obstetrical operations. Spinal anaesthesia is clearly easier to perform, provides a greater depth of conduction blockade and thus may be more

Table 5.5. Cardiovascular response (% change) to equal sensory levels of spinal and epidural anaesthesia. Reproduced with permission from Ward et al.[22]

	Spinal	Epidural without epinephrine	Epidural with epinephrine
Mean arterial blood pressure	-21.3	-8.9	-22.0
Pulse rate	+3.7	+6.7	+15.8
Cardiac output	-17.7	-5.4	+30.2
Stroke volume	-25.4	-10.2	+7.9
Total peripheral vascular resistance	-5.0	-2.9	-39.6

useful for surgical patients. On the other hand, continuous epidural analgesia is preferable for prolonged pain relief, due to the lower incidence of post-spinal headache, reduced haemodynamic depression and the ability to achieve more effective separation of sensory and motor blockade.

Spinal anaesthesia for surgical operations

Spinal anaesthesia produces intense blockade of those spinal nerves, and the spinal cord, which are exposed to the injected local anaesthetic. Somatic pain and motor function are abolished in the blocked segments. Visceral pain is also prevented if the appropriate afferent nerves are blocked. The sympathetic system which derives from the spinal segments T1-L2 is also affected to varying degrees, depending on the height of the blockade.

The sacral parasympathetic afferent nerves arising from the pelvic viscera are blocked in virtually all cases. However, the main parasympathetic nerve, the vagus, is a cranial nerve, and is unaffected by spinal anaesthesia. Its contribution to visceral pain is pro-

Table 5.6. The surgical procedures that can be performed under spinal anaesthesia.

Operation	Suitability of spinal blockade	Height of block required	Remarks
Lower abdominal	+++	T7	Reduced bleeding.
Caesarean section	+++	T6	Must avoid aortocaval occlusion. May require IV opioid after delivery.
Urological (transurethral)	+++	T9 - 10	
Open operation on kidney	++	T6	May need artificial ventilation if pleural cavity opened.
Vaginal	+++	T10-12	Reduced bleeding. May need higher block if peritoneum opened.
Perineal including anal and rectal	+++	T12	
Lower limbs	+++	T12	Reduced deep venous thrombosis. Continuous technique very suitable for the elderly.
Upper abdominal	+ / -	T5	Unblocked vagus can cause problems unless patient paralysed and ventilated.

bably minimal because its afferent fibres mostly mediate the sensations of hunger and nausea. It is important to remember that because the vagus nerve remains unblocked, a vasovagal reaction can occur in some patients.

Postoperatively, analgesia will last only as long as the local anaesthetic drug is effective, and will be accompanied by paralysis of the lower limbs.

Indications

Spinal anaesthesia may be used for all surgical procedures involving the abdomen, the perineum and the lower limbs. Since spinal anaesthesia is mainly performed using a single injection, its use is usually restricted to operations that can be completed within the duration of that single injection. Therefore it is particularly useful for urological procedures, herniorrhaphy and operations on the lower limb (Table 5.6).

Contraindications

There are few absolute contraindications to spinal anaesthesia. Each case should be decided on its merits and the risk/benefit assessed. Obvious contraindications, such as sepsis of the skin at the lumbar puncture site and allergy to local anaesthetic drugs, are extremely rare. Other conditions which must be considered are:

Hypovolaemic shock

Patients whose arterial pressure is being maintained by intense vasoconstriction are very susceptible to rapid and possibly disastrous hypotension when the spinal anaesthesia starts to affect the sympathetic outflow. Nevertheless, in many patients, adequate preoperative resuscitation is usually possible if haemorrhage is not present and continuing. If the priority is to stop the bleeding by surgical intervention, then spinal anaesthesia is best avoided. If haemorrhage is not the cause of the hypovolaemia, it is usually possible to rehydrate under careful monitoring, to the point when spinal anaesthesia could be a good choice, e.g. for a strangulated inguinal hernia or a fractured neck of femur.

Septicaemia or bacteraemia

Meningitis and/or epidural abscess following spinal anaesthesia is extremely rare even in the presence of septicaemia or bacteraemia.[24,25] Most cases of epidural abscess have involved a blood-borne organism presumably colonizing a haematoma, but such cases also occur spontaneously without a spinal or epidural injection.[25]

Pre-existing neurological disease

Once considered an absolute contraindication, there is now considerable evidence that a central nerve block is most unlikely to exacerbate pre-existing diseases such as multiple sclerosis.

Increased intracranial pressure

Lumbar puncture is a risk in such patients.

Haemorrhagic diathesis

Severe cases usually preclude surgery in any event. However, there has been much discussion on the wisdom of using spinal or epidural block with the current practice of mini-heparinization, and a large body of opinion believes that this is not a contraindication. Spinal puncture is generally considered less traumatic than epidural cannulation and catheterization, but both techniques can damage blood vessels. In cases of doubt a simple coagulation test will show if the heparin has had an abnormally excessive effect on blood clotting. A full coagulation screen is advisable in some cases.

It has been suggested that intraoperative heparinization, low dose heparin and aspirin therapy could be hazardous in spinal anaesthesia, but surveys have shown that the problem is more theoretical than real.[26-29]

Patient refusal

This must be handled sympathetically and intelligently, especially if there is a particular need to use spinal anaesthesia.

Management of surgical patients during spinal anaesthesia

Preoperative assessment

As with all forms of anaesthesia, a preoperative visit is essential not only to examine the patient but to describe and explain the anaesthetic procedure. While most patients will accept the judgement of the anaesthesiologist as to what is best for them, some have reservations about spinal anaesthesia and they need reassurance. Some are unwilling to remain awake during surgery, and in most cases sedation or a concomitant general anaesthetic can be offered. If it is important for reluctant patients to be awake, then they must be persuaded of the advantages. It is wrong to insist on a particular method of anaesthesia if patients remain adamant that they do not want it and there is no indication for it.

The attitude of the whole surgical team is important to success if patients are to remain awake. Nurses, surgeons and anaesthesiologists must be sympathetic and supportive, and refrain from making remarks which can alarm the patient. The surgeon must work with reasonable gentleness and speed. Should the patient experience discomfort or anxiety, the anaesthesiologist must be able to give reassurance and administer analgesics and/or sedatives.

Premedication

This is usually given an hour before surgery and the oral or intramuscular routes are the most commonly used. Personal preference dictates whether an opioid or a sedative or both is used. An opioid will reduce discomfort during performance of the block.

Sedatives and analgesics

Intraoperative medication is frequently required because the patient is either nervous and/or uncomfortable. Anxiolytics are widely used with regional anaesthesia. They are effective in producing a calm, sleepy and compliant patient. However, they have no analgesic properties and should not be used alone in a patient complaining of pain. The benzodiazepines, e.g. diazepam, temazepam and midazolam, are usually given in divided intravenous doses until the required sedation is achieved. They have relatively long half-lives and are potent amnesics. They are also respiratory depressants.[30,31]

Sedation with short-acting hypnotic drugs, such as thiopental, methohexitone, propofol and chlormethiazole (not available in the USA), given by intravenous infusion, is also used. The sedation may be light or deep as required and recovery is usually rapid when the infusion is stopped.

Opioids are the drugs of choice if the patient's main complaint is pain or discomfort. Again, divided doses given intravenously until the patient is comfortable give the best results. All the common opioids have sedative properties, but they can also cause nausea and vomiting, and respiratory depression. Ketamine is an alternative to opioids preferred by some.

Concomitant general anaesthesia

The combination of spinal blockade and light general anaesthesia is an excellent form of balanced anaesthesia, with a wide range of indications.[32-35] It can be used for operations that are inappropriate with conscious patients, such as those in the upper abdomen. It has the following advantages:

1. The patient often prefers to be asleep, particularly during long operations.

2. Any pain from a less than perfect block is not felt by the patient.

3. The constraints imposed on the surgical team by the patient remaining conscious are avoided.

4. If induced hypotension is indicated to minimize blood loss[35], the arterial pressure can be readily reduced by increasing the depth of the general anaesthesia. Conscious patients tolerate hypotension badly.

5. If a full general anaesthetic becomes necessary (e.g. an unexpectedly lengthy operation, or one extending beyond the blocked segments), this is easy to achieve without upset to the patient or the surgical team. Patients should always be prepared for the possibility of a general anaesthetic, planned or unplanned.

It is important to remember that the general anaesthesia should be as light and as simple as possible. It is not required to provide either muscle relaxation or analgesia, unless the spinal block is partially ineffective. It is frequently not necessary to intubate the trachea, since a mask anaesthetic, with an oral or laryngeal airway, allows a lighter plane of anaesthesia than is the case with an endotracheal tube. However, intubation of the patient is left to the discretion of the anaesthesiologist.

Controlled ventilation is not required for the vast majority of operations performed under combined spinal and general anaesthesia and spontaneous breathing has much to recommend it. For example:

(a) relaxants are not required, (b) the patient cannot become awake without it being obvious, (c) the adequacy of the spinal blockade is easily judged, (d) an accidental disconnection on the anaesthetic machine will be quickly evident and will not cause a disaster, and (e) observation of the reservoir bag clearly indicates gaseous exchange in the lungs, and the adequacy of respiration can be easily measured with oximetry and capnography.

Perioperative management

Monitoring of the heart rate, arterial pressure and ECG are essential. Unconscious patients must also be observed in regard to their airway and breathing. Quiet regular breathing indicates that the patient has a satisfactory block and is asleep. Apnoea may be due to too light a plane of anaesthesia, obstructed airway, respiratory depression or circulatory arrest. Where available oximetry and/or capnography should be used.[36-38]

Hypotension

Hypotension should be treated promptly unless it is induced to reduce bleeding. Preloading the patient with 500-1000 mL of crystalloid solution is frequently employed to prevent hypotension. To treat hypotension, it is better to use a vasopressor drug (e.g. ephedrine 5-15 mg) which produces a rapid effect (sometimes it requires more than one injection) regardless of whether the hypotension is due to sympathetic blockade, vasovagal fainting or both. Alternatively a drug such as phenylephrine can be given by I.V. infusion, the dose being titrated to the patient's blood pressure response. Hypotension is discussed in detail on p. 150. If haemorrhage occurs during surgery, it can cause marked hypotension in the presence of widespread sympathetic blockade. It should be treated without delay, using fluids, plasma and blood as necessary. Raising the blood pressure with a vasoconstrictor under these circumstances is not appropriate.

Induced hypotension

Because hypotension is poorly tolerated in conscious patients, hypotensive spinal anaesthesia given to reduce blood loss should only be used in combination with general anaesthesia.[32-34] It is especially indicated in radical surgery involving considerable blood loss (radical hysterectomy, abdomino-perineal resection of the rectum, etc.) but is also useful in less major operations (e.g. vaginal repairs) where even small amounts of blood can obscure the operative field.

The technique depends upon the combination of spinal anaesthesia and deep general anaesthesia. The arterial pressure seldom decreases to a sufficiently low level with light general anaesthesia and increasing the concentration of a potent volatile agent may be necessary.[34] The level of hypotension should be judged by the amount of bleeding in the operative site. Spinal anaesthesia can reduce blood loss in many operations without hypotension (see p. 129).

Postoperative management

Patients who have had spinal anaesthesia usually regain their mental faculties quickly if deep sedation is avoided. Even when general anaesthesia has been added, the patient awakens quickly and recovers all reflexes necessary for maintenance of the airway, usually before the onset of postoperative pain.

The blood pressure tends to be labile for an hour or so after surgery, though hypotension seldom causes any problem. If the pressure is considered too low, it may be increased quickly and easily. Raising the foot of the bed prevents pooling of blood in dependent veins. The intravenous infusion of 250-500 mL crystalloid given over 15-30 min often increases the arterial pressure to acceptable levels. In severe cases or when a rapid response is required, a vasopressor, e.g. ephedrine (5-15 mg), may be given intravenously and repeated if necessary. An intramuscular injection of ephedrine (25-50 mg) at the same time as the intravenous dose will maintain the pressure over a longer period.

It is unusual to have to resort to vasopressors in a patient more than once. Indeed, in such cases an alternative cause for the hypotension, such as haemorrhage, should be sought.

As the legs may remain numb and paralysed for some time, the patient should be reassured that recovery will be complete. Attention to pressure points with changes in posture may be required if the block is prolonged.

Spinal anaesthesia in obstetrics

Until recent years, epidural rather than spinal blockade has been used in obstetrics. However, many anaesthesiologists are now finding spinal anaesthesia particularly useful for Caesarean section. The more rapid onset and more profound anaesthesia produced by spinal blockade are its main advantages.

In cases of urgency, spinal anaesthesia has much to offer, avoiding as it does the inherent dangers of general anaesthesia in a mother with a potentially full stomach, and in whom the relatively long onset time of an epidural could jeopardize the foetus. With a spinal block, most mothers will be ready for operation within 5-10 min of making the injection. While some clinicians have concern about the rapid onset of sympathetic blockade, this should not be a particular problem if the mother is kept in the lateral position, and if the arterial pressure is adequately monitored and hypotension promptly treated with ephedrine.

For the relief of pain in labour, epidural block is indisputably superior to spinal block because it is easier to produce a differential nerve block with the former. However, there is one situation in which a continuous spinal might be used for analgesia, namely accidental dural tap. Dural tap occurs in about 0.5-1% of mothers receiving epidural analgesia. The usual practice is to remove the needle and attempt to find the epidural space at an adjacent intervertebral space. However, this can lead to considerable confusion, as cerebrospinal fluid leaking into the epidural space can find its way down the reinserted needle, thus mimicking a second dural tap. Also there is uncertainty in such cases about whether, and how much, local anaesthetic can reach the subarachnoid space. It seems more logical to insert the catheter into the subarachnoid space and reduce the amount of local anaesthetic appropriately.[39,40] 1-1.5 mL of 0.5% plain bupivacaine will suffice in most mothers.

Caesarean section

Preparation

When explaining spinal anaesthesia to the mother it is important not to promise total analgesia during the operation. While this will be achieved in most patients, some will experience a degree of discomfort or pain, and the anaesthesiologist should explain how it will be relieved (vide infra). Unfulfilled promises can have a bad effect upon the patient's morale. The possibility of a postoperative headache should also be mentioned.

Height of block

Most authorities put the desired height of block for Caesarean section around T4-T6. The evidence for this is slight, however, as one may see a completely painless section with a block to T9 and a degree of pain even with a block to T2. Pain during a Caesarean section is invariably due to visceral pain arising from the uterus, the bladder or the peritoneum, and it is probably the intensity of the nerve blockade rather than its height which is of greater importance.

Because the pregnant patient is more sensitive to the effects of local anaesthetics (p. 94), she is usually given a reduced amount for spinal anaesthesia. The most commonly used drugs are hyperbaric lidocaine, bupivacaine and tetracaine. Doses that provide good operating conditions are: lidocaine, 75 mg; bupivacaine and tetracaine, 12.5 mg. If lidocaine is used, the operation should not last longer than 45-60 min. Isobaric bupivacaine (15 mg) is also used for spinal anaesthesia for Caesarean section.[41] The quality of anaesthesia and analgesia is improved when fentanyl (10 $\mu g \cdot mL^{-1}$) is added to the local anaesthetic[42] (see p. 101).

Hypotension

Because the uterine blood flow is dependent upon arterial pressure, hypotension is poorly tolerated by the foetus. The circulatory changes occurring during late pregnancy and delivery, and the added effects of spinal anaesthesia, are complex. Hypotension may be sudden and profound and can occur at any time from the injection of the local anaesthetic to the delivery. Hypotension after delivery is uncommon unless there is significant bleeding.

Hypotension may be caused by sympathetic blockade, inferior vena caval (IVC) occlusion or haemorrhage. Hypertension may result at delivery from relief of IVC occlusion, excessive dosage of vasopressors, and the elimination of the placental circulation enhancing the increased blood volume and cardiac output present in late pregnancy.[43]

The administration of substantial volumes of fluid, both electrolyte or colloid, to prevent hypotension is an almost universal practice. However, the evidence for its efficacy is meagre and the failure rate (as judged by the necessity to use a vasopressor) is substantial (25-60% in most published studies).[44] This is hardly surprising as it is unlikely that otherwise healthy mothers will be dehydrated at the time of Caesarean section, and the increase in blood volume and cardiac output caused by the fluid load is of short duration.[45]

Prevention of IVC occlusion is important and the avoidance of the supine posture is necessary until the baby is delivered. While a wedge maintaining a semilateral tilt to the left should be used during the initial surgery, it should be remembered that IVC occlusion may still be present in this position. During the onset of spinal anaesthesia, it is wiser to use a complete lateral tilt. Since this can lead to a unilateral block, it is best to perform the spinal injection on one side, and then turn the patient to the opposite side after injection.

Treatment

The essential trigger to the development of hypotension is sympathetic blockade resulting in widespread vasodilatation. This can cause hypotension by itself, but in late pregnancy it will in addition "reveal" IVC occlusion, i.e. it reverses the vasoconstriction by which many mothers maintain a normal arterial pressure in the presence of total or partial IVC occlusion.[43] Lastly sympathetic blockade can lead to severe hypotension with sudden bradycardia and syncope.

A vasopressor is therefore the most logical form of treatment. If agents known to cause a decrease in uterine blood flow (e.g. methoxamine) are avoided, the hypotension will be rapidly reversed, together with the symptoms and signs of vagal overactivity if present. The only danger is overdosage, which may not become obvious until after the delivery, when IVC occlusion is totally relieved and there is a dramatic decrease in uterine blood flow.

The arterial pressure and pulse rate must be closely observed after the spinal injection and any decrease should be treated rapidly.[46] The choice of vasopressor is a personal one (see p. 152), but the use of an IV infusion rather than repeated bolus injections has much to recommend it. However, intermittent injections of 5-10 mg of ephedrine are considered by many to be the treatment of choice. Atropine is not a good choice (see p. 62) even in the presence of marked bradycardia.

Vaginal delivery

The use of a spinal saddle block for the later stages of a vaginal delivery was widely practised, particularly in North America. It allows a painless delivery, with or without instrumentation, and the performance and repair of an episiotomy. To relieve the pain of uterine contractions, however, the block must reach T10.

Lumbar puncture is performed with the patient sitting. A small quantity of local anaesthetic, e.g. 0.5-1 mL of 0.5% hyperbaric bupivacaine, is injected and the patient is kept sitting for a few minutes until perineal anaesthesia develops.

Retained placenta

Spinal anaesthesia is frequently preferred to general anaesthesia for removal of a retained placenta, provided blood loss has not been severe.

Paediatric spinal anaesthesia

Spinal anaesthesia is used mainly in preterm infants who survive the early neonatal period and require surgery below the umbilicus, because these infants are prone to develop life-threatening apnoea and/or bradycardia after general anaesthesia. A randomized blinded trial showed that unsupplemented spinal anaesthesia in infants who had been born preterm produced no postoperative apnoeic episodes with bradycardia, compared to 31% in infants who received general anaesthesia, and 89% in those given sedation with IM ketamine (1-2 $mg \cdot kg^{-1}$) prior to induction of spinal anaesthesia.[47]

Abajian et al[48], were the first to report using spinal anaesthesia for surgery in the high-risk infant. Infants not maintained on intravenous feeding are allowed a normal oral intake up to 4 h before surgery and are premedicated with IM atropine (0.02 $mg \cdot kg^{-1}$). The electrocardiogram, heart and breath sounds, blood pressure and oxygen saturation should be monitored. Application of the blood pressure cuff to the anaesthetized lower extremity diminishes arousal of the infant during surgery. With the monitors attached, the infant is placed in the lateral decubitus position with its chin extended. Chin extension optimizes airway management and therefore oxygenation during lumbar puncture in infants.[48] After a free flow of cerebrospinal fluid is obtained, a 1 mL insulin syringe is used to administer the local anaesthetic. The doses used for spinal anaesthesia in infants[49] are shown in Table 5.7.

After removal of the spinal needle, the infant is placed in the supine position and the legs observed for signs of paralysis, which usually occurs within 2 min. An intravenous infusion is then started in the anaesthetized foot or ankle. This avoids upsetting the child before the lumbar puncture is performed. Although induction of spinal anaesthesia before starting an IV infusion is controversial, this is the generally accepted practice since spinal anaesthesia in infants causes little change in blood pressure or pulse rate.[48]

While not widely employed in older paediatric patients, spinal anaesthesia can be used with advantage for operations of short duration (45-60 min) in neonates and young premature infants. It is suitable for operations such as inguinal hernia repair and for surgery of the external genitalia and lower extremities. The complete limb paralysis produced by spinal anaesthesia greatly facilitates the surgical management of these infants who receive no general anaesthesia. Spinal anaesthesia in neonates and infants can be of surprisingly short duration even with a long-acting local anaesthetic. [48,50,51]

Table 5.7. Choice of local anaesthetic in infants based on anticipated duration of operation[48]

Duration (min)	Drug	Diluent	Dose ($mg \cdot kg^{-1}$)
30	Lidocaine 5%	Dextrose 7.5%/epineprine	3.0
60	Tetracaine 0.5%	Dextrose 5%	0.4
60	Bupivacaine 0.75%	Dextrose 8.25%	3.0
90	Tetracaine 0.5%	Dextrose 5%/epineprine	0.4

Dose of epinephrine is aproximately 50$\mu g \cdot mL^{-1}$

Pain therapy

Subarachnoid injection can be used to provide prolonged pain relief, particularly in patients with cancer. Three distinct possibilities are available: (a) repeated injection, or continuous infusion of, an opioid, (b) spinal nerve destruction using a neurolytic agent such as phenol or alcohol, and (c) transcutaneous cordotomy using high frequency diathermy.

Intrathecal opioids

Intrathecal opioids are now established in the treatment of cancer pain which cannot be adequately controlled by simpler methods of opioid administration.[52,53] The ability to produce segmental analgesia without nerve blockade is a considerable advantage. Because a much lower dose is required with intrathecal compared to epidural injection, it is especially suitable for implanted injection devices.[54]

Respiratory depression is unlikely in patients who are, or have recently been, receiving large doses of oral or parenteral opioid.

For continuous infusions, the dose of morphine is 0.5 mg in 24 h, increasing if necessary up to 2.0 mg in 24 h. Other opioids such as fentanyl or its derivatives can be used in equipotent doses.

Intrathecal neurolysis

Intrathecal neurolysis can relieve pain for prolonged periods in terminally ill patients. The objective is to destroy the nerves subserving the pain, without affecting adjacent nerves, and limiting the effect as much as possible to the posterior spinal nerve roots.
The risk of seriously compromising sphincter control by destroying autonomic nerves is ever-present. Each patient presents an individual problem and neurolytic procedures should only be contemplated when other methods of pain relief have been explored and found wanting. The most commonly used agents are alcohol (hypobaric) and phenol (hyperbaric). For techniques and dosages consult specialist textbooks.[55]

Transcutaneous cordotomy

Transcutaneous cordotomy is an elegant technique for relieving cancer pain.[56] Under radiological control the spinal cord in the neck is visualized after the intrathecal injection of contrast medium. The posterior spinothalamic tracts are stimulated electrically, producing a sensation of hot or cold or paraesthesia on the contralateral side. Once the appropriate spinal tracts involved in the pain are identified, they are destroyed by thermocoagulation. The best results are obtained in patients with unilateral pain and in most cases, only patients with a limited prognosis should be considered for this technique.

Drugs and dosage

The local anaesthetic drugs used for spinal anaesthesia are fully described on pp. 84 and 97.

Spinal anaesthesia is unique in that a small amount of drug rapidly produces a wide band of anaesthesia. The dose required is only about 10% of that needed for an epidural block, and systemic toxicity is of no concern.

However, many factors affect the spread of the drug once it has been injected into the subarachnoid space[57], and individual variations can be wide. Although in recent years many of these factors have been studied and quantified, the clinician wants an answer to the question "How much of what drug do I inject into this patient for this operation?" In spite of our increasing knowledge of how spinal anaesthesia may be varied by such things as dosage, baricity, posture, site of lumbar puncture, patient age and weight, etc., a pragmatic approach still has much to recommend it. The anaesthesiologist must try to anaesthetize 100% of his patients, and to do this, many patients will receive a greater dose than is strictly required.[58] One must be prepared for the consequences of this, namely an unduly high blockade and/or hypotension. Conversely, the occurrence of an occasional inadequate block must be faced and a strategy worked out in advance.

However, spinal anaesthesia can be manipulated to a certain extent by:

The choice of drug

As all the drugs commonly used for spinal anaesthesia produce rapid and profound nerve blockade, the choice of drug is based on the expected duration of the operation.

The dose injected

The total dose is more important than volume or concentration. As mentioned on p. 86, the relationship between dosage and height of block is not linear.[59] Varying the volume between 2-4 mL of the same concentration of drug may produce little difference in the height of block. At the injection site in the lumbar region, the whole cauda equina (L1-S5) is available to the drug, but to reach the upper thoracic segments, the drug must ascend a considerable distance (Fig. 1.24, p. 27). Moreover the drugs spread laterally into the dural cuffs of the spinal nerves, as well as cephalad. Thus a larger dose may affect the nerves over a longer segment of their intrathecal length, giving rise to a longer duration of block rather than a more widespread block. This explains the well-documented observation that increasing dosage prolongs the anaesthesia rather than increasing the height of blockade.[60]

Baricity and gravity

With small volume injections and using gravity at its maximum, i.e. with the patient sitting up, it is possible to make the local anaesthetic spread caudad with a hyperbaric solution or cephalad with a hypobaric solution.

With larger volumes, however, it is more difficult to manipulate the height of block in this way. With the patient lying in the Trendelenburg position or turned laterally, the initial spread may be affected, but once the patient is turned supine and horizontal, the eventual spread is only marginally different.[61] Thus a unilateral block can be obtained using a hyperbaric solution with the patient kept in the lateral position, but it will soon become bilateral when the supine position is resumed.[61]

Perhaps more interesting is the difference in behaviour between hyperbaric and isobaric solutions when gravity is not used, i.e. the patient is kept horizontal throughout.[62] Hyperbaric solutions invariably produce higher blocks than isobaric solutions and it is difficult to ensure a mid-thoracic block with isobaric solutions unless large volumes (4-5 mL) are used.[62] The greater ability of hyperbaric solutions to reach more cephalad nerves may have more to do with their lower miscibility than their baricity. Thus the injectate remains unmixed with CSF for a longer time, promoting increased spread. In any event, an isobaric solution is excellent for lower limb surgery, particularly in the elderly, in whom a very high block is unnecessary and undesirable, while a hyperbaric solution is more suitable for abdominal surgery.[57]

Patient characteristics

Age, sex and weight may be largely discounted as factors which influence the subarachnoid spread of local anaesthetic solutions.[57] Height, on the other hand, should, on basic principles, have some effect as in a tall individual the drug has further to go to achieve the same cephalad spread. However, there are no convincing data on which an appropriate allowance can be made for the patient's height.[57,59] The most likely cause for this is that the length of the spinal column is much less variable than the height of individuals. Excessively tall or short people owe their stature in the main to the length of their lower limbs. In any event the height of 90% of the population, including both men and women, only varies by about 17% (1.56 m to 1.82 m), and making an adjustment in dosage of this magnitude to allow for height borders on pedantry.

Needle position and method of injection

Virtually all subarachnoid injections will be made through the 4 intervertebral spaces from L2/3 to L5/S1. Thus, with few exceptions,[63] the interspace used has little effect on the spread of spinal anaesthesia.[57]

Whether the needle bevel is pointing cephalad, caudad or lateral could make a small difference with larger needles but probably has no effect on spread with the smaller needles now in use.

Barbotage was popular when large needles were used, but it is virtually impossible to perform with smal-bore needles, as the repeated aspiration and reinjection takes too long.

Addition of vasoconstrictor drugs

In other forms of regional anaesthesia, vasoconstrictors increase duration by reducing absorption of local anaesthetic from the site of injection.

Vasoconstrictors, particularly epinephrine and phenylephrine, can also increase the duration of spinal anaesthesia (p. 87), though their mode of action is not clear. A reduction in blood flow in the capillaries responsible for absorbing local anaesthetic in the structures within the subarachnoid space has not been demonstrated, and indeed could be a potential hazard if it does occur. Other possible mechanisms include the lowering of pH due to the addition of the vasoconstrictor, or the modulation of neural activity in descending spinal pathways involved in nociception.[64] The clinician must ask whether their addition is going to be clinically significant in a given patient. While controlled, double-blind trials show that spinal blockade is prolonged by adding vasoconstrictors, the degree of prolongation varies considerably.[65-71] Thus the prolongation is considered of little clinical value with bupivacaine[70] and lidocaine[69], but useful with tetracaine.[71] Even those who claim considerable prolongation have found a large individual variation, and some patients can have a longer block with a plain solution than others with a vasoconstrictor.

Although variable in its effect in prolonging the useful duration of spinal anaesthesia, addition of a vasoconstrictor drug usually increases the time for complete recovery in the lumbar and sacral regions, prolonging the recovery room stay.

Guidelines for use of local anaesthetic solutions

Operations can be arbitrarily categorized as those requiring nerve blockade above or below the first lumbar (L1) dermatome (Table 5.8).

Above L1

1. Herniorrhaphy
2. Intra-abdominal surgery
3. Genitourinary operations (transurethral resection, cystoscopy and operations on the bladder neck)
4. Gynaecological operations requiring a T10 dermatome level (D&C, cerclage, cone biopsy)
5. Caesarean section

A hyperbaric solution is recommended for these procedures. These solutions gravitate to the T4-6 level in the supine patient, assuring an adequate level of analgesia.

Below L1

1. Lower limb orthopaedic operations (including the hip)
2. Genitourinary operations (penile implant, and urethral operations below the membranous urethra)
3. Perineal operations
4. Lower limb vascular operations (femoral-popliteal bypass graft)
5. Amputations of the lower limbs
6. Rectal operations
7. Vaginal delivery

For these operations an isobaric solution which tends to remain at lower dermatomes, providing intense anaesthesia of prolonged duration is recommended. However, hyperbaric solutions can be used but may cause unnecessarily high blocks unless positioning is used to limit cephalad spread.

Hyperbaric solutions

1. **Procaine** 10% (a 5% solution can be prepared by diluting 1:1 with 10% dextrose, normal saline or distilled water)
2. **Lidocaine** 5%, dextrose 7.5% (manufactured premixed)
3. **Mepivacaine** 4%, dextrose 9.25% (manufactured premixed)
4. **Bupivacaine** 0.75%, dextrose 8.25% or 0.5% in dextrose 8% (manufactured premixed)
5. **Tetracaine** 0.5%, dextrose 5%, (mix equal volumes of 1% tetracaine and 10% dextrose)
6. **Cinchocaine** 0.5%, dextrose 6% (available in some countries)

Isobaric solutions

1. **Lidocaine** 2%
2. **Bupivacaine** 0.5% or 0.75%
3. **Tetracaine** 0.5% (mix equal volume of 1% tetracaine and preservative-free normal saline or CSF)
4. **Cinchocaine** 0.5% (available in some countries)

Local anaesthetic solutions employed for isobaric spinal anaesthesia should **not** contain preservatives or antioxidants such as methylparaben, sodium sulphite or sodium metabisulphite.

Hypobaric solutions

1. **Bupivacaine** 0.25% (1:1 dilution of 0.5% plain bupivacaine with distilled water)
2. **Tetracaine** 0.1-0.33% (1mL of 1% tetracaine diluted to 3-10 mL with distilled water. Alternatively, dilute tetracaine niphanoid crystals to a final concentration of 0.1-0.33% with distilled water)
3. **Cinchocaine** 0.067% (available in some countries)

Although hypobaric solutions are utilized for operations below the L1 dermatome, operations in these regions can be carried out equally well with an isobaric solution.

Hypobaric solutions are usually reserved for rectal, perineal and lower extremity operations done with the patient in the lateral decubitus or prone jack-knife position with a head-down tilt.

Table 5.8. Guidelines for the employment of local anaesthetic solutions in spinal anaesthesia

Block height	Solution	conc (%)	Total* dose (mg)	Usual volume (mL)	Approx. duration** no epi*** (min)	Approx. duration** 0.2mg epi*** (min)****
Above L1	**Hyperbaric**					
	Procaine	5.0	100-200	2-4	30-60	-
	Lidocaine	5.0	50-100	1-2	45-90	45-90
	Bupivacaine	0.5	15	3	90-180	90-180
	Mepivacaine	4.0	40-100	1-2.5	45-90	45-90
	Bupivacaine	0.75	15	2	90-180	90-180
	Tetracaine	0.5	15	3	90-180	90-180
	Cinchocaine	0.5	10	2	90-180	90-180
Below L1	**Isobaric**					
	Lidocaine	2.0	60	3	60-120	90-150
	Mepivacaine	2.0	60	3	60-120	90-150
	Bupivacaine	0.5	15	3	90-240	240-300
	Tetracaine	0.5	15	3	90-240	240-300
	Cinchocaine	0.5	15	3	90-240	240-300
	Hypobaric					
	Bupivacaine	0.25	7.5-10	3-4	90-240	-
	Tetracaine	0.1-0.33	4-10	4-10	90-240	-
	Cinchocaine	0.067	3-7	5-10	90-240	-

* Although a dose range is given, the larger amounts are recommended to improve the quality of block and likelihood of success (p. 142)
** Duration of surgical anaesthesia
*** Epinephrine
**** See sections on vasoconstrictors p. 87 and 143. Epinephrine does not appear to prolong anaesthesia in the thoracic dermatomes. Some prolongation is observed in the lumbosacral regions. The prolongation shown here is merely an estimate of what may occur and is not necessarily experimentally determined.

Isobaric solutions of bupivacaine and lidocaine are not approved by the FDA for spinal anaesthesia. However, this use has been reported in numerous publications. Solutions used for spinal anaesthesia should **not** contain any preservatives or antioxidants such as methylparaben, sodium sulphite or sodium metabisulphite.

Adapted with permission, Lambert and Covino[72]

49. Rice LJ (1988) Regional anesthesia in pediatrics. In ASA 39th annual refresher course lectures and clinical update program. Illinois: American Society of Anesthesiologists 123

50. Saint-Maurice C (1990) Spinal block. In: Saint-Maurice C, Schulte-Steinberg 0 ed. Regional anesthesia in children. Fribourg, Switzerland: Mediglobe, 123

51. Parkinson SK, Little WL, Malley RA, Pecsok JL, Mueller JB, Whalen T (1990). Use of hyperbaric bupivacaine with epinephrine for spinal anesthesia in infants. Reg Anesth 15:86

52. Cousins MJ, Cherry DA, Gourlay GK (1988) Acute and chronic pain: use of spinal opiods. In: Cousins M, Bridenbaugh P ed. Neural blockade. Philadelphia: JB Lippincott, Co., 1006

53. Coombs DW, Maurer LH, Saunders RL, Gaylor M (1984) Outcomes and complications of intraspinal narcotic analgesia for cancer pain control. J Clin Oncol 2:1414

54. Penn RD, Paice JA, Gottschalk W, Ivankovich AD (1984) Cancer pain relief using chronic morphine infusion. Early experience with a programmable implanted drug pump. J Neurosurg 61:302

55. Bonica JJ, Buckley FP, Moricca G, Murphy TM (1990) Neurolytic blockage and hypophysectomy. In: Bonica J ed. The management of pain. Philadelphia: Lea & Febiger, 1991

56. Rosomoff HL, Papo I, Loeser JD, Bonica JJ (1990) Neurosurgical operations on the spinal cord. In: Bonica J ed. The management of pain. Philadelphia: Lea & Febiger, 2067

57. Greene NM (1985) Distribution of local anesthetic solutions within the subarachnoid space. Anesth Analg 64:715

58. Lambert DH (1989) Factors influencing spinal anesthesia. Int Anesthesiol Clin 27:13

59. Norris MC (1988) Height, weight, and the spread of subarachnoid hyperbaric bupivacaine in the term parturient. Anesth Analg 67:555

60. Sheskey MC, Rocco AG, Bizzarri-Schmid M, Francis DM, Edström H, Covino BG (1983) A dose-response study of bupivacaine for spinal anesthesia. Anesth Analg 62:931

61. Wildsmith JA, McClure JH, Brown DT, Scott DB (1981) Effect of posture on the spread of isobaric and hyperbaric amethocaine. Br J Anaesth 53:273

62. Brown DT, Wildsmith JA, Covino BG, Scott DB (1980) Effects of baricity on spinal anaesthesia with amethocaine. Br J Anaesth 52:589

63. Tuominen M, Taivainen T, Rosenberg PH (1989) Spread of spinal anesthesia with plain bupivacaine: influence of the vertebral interspace used for injection. BR J Anaesth 62:358

64. Collins JG, Kitahata LM, Matsumoto M (1984) Spinally administered epinephrine suppresses noxiously evoked activity of WDR neurons in the dorsal horn of the spinal cord. Anesthesiology 60:269

65 Vaida GT, Moss P, Capan LM, Turndoff H (1986) Prolongation of lidocaine spinal anesthesia with phenylephrine. Anesth Analg 65:781

66. Lawrence VS, Rich CR, Magitzky L, Lee JH (1984) Spinal anesthesia with isobaric lidocaine 2% and the effect of phenylephrine. Reg Anesth 9:17

67. Racle JP, Benkhadra A, Poy JY, Gleizal B (1987) Effects of increasing amounts of epinephrine during isobaric spinal anesthesia in elderly patients. Anesth Analg 66:882

68. Meagher RP, Moore DC, DeVries JC (1966) Phenylephrine: the most effective potentiator of tetracaine spinal anesthesia. Anesth Analg 45:134

69. Chambers WA, Littlewood DG, Logan MR, Scott DB (1982) Effect of added epineprine on spinal anesthesia with lidocaine. Anesth Analg 60:417

70. Chambers WA, Littlewood DG, Scott DB (1982) Spinal anesthesia with hyperbaric bupivacaine: effect of added vasoconstrictors. Anesth Analg 61:49

71. Armstrong IR, Littlewood DG, Chambers WA (1983) Spinal anesthesia with tetracaine - effect of added vasoconstrictors. Anesth Analg 62:793

72. Lambert DH, Covino BG (1987) Hyperbaric, hypobaric and isobaric spinal anesthesia. Res Staff Phys 33:79

Hypobaric solutions

1. **Bupivacaine** 0.25% (1:1 dilution of 0.5% plain bupivacaine with distilled water)
2. **Tetracaine** 0.1-0.33% (1mL of 1% tetracaine diluted to 3-10 mL with distilled water. Alternatively, dilute tetracaine niphanoid crystals to a final concentration of 0.1-0.33% with distilled water)
3. **Cinchocaine** 0.067% (available in some countries)

Although hypobaric solutions are utilized for operations below the L1 dermatome, operations in these regions can be carried out equally well with an isobaric solution.

Hypobaric solutions are usually reserved for rectal, perineal and lower extremity operations done with the patient in the lateral decubitus or prone jack-knife position with a head-down tilt.

Table 5.8. Guidelines for the employment of local anaesthetic solutions in spinal anaesthesia

Block height	Solution	conc (%)	Total* dose (mg)	Usual volume (mL)	Approx. duration** no epi*** (min)	Approx. duration** 0.2mg epi*** (min)****
Above L1	**Hyperbaric**					
	Procaine	5.0	100-200	2-4	30-60	-
	Lidocaine	5.0	50-100	1-2	45-90	45-90
	Bupivacaine	0.5	15	3	90-180	90-180
	Mepivacaine	4.0	40-100	1-2.5	45-90	45-90
	Bupivacaine	0.75	15	2	90-180	90-180
	Tetracaine	0.5	15	3	90-180	90-180
	Cinchocaine	0.5	10	2	90-180	90-180
Below L1	**Isobaric**					
	Lidocaine	2.0	60	3	60-120	90-150
	Mepivacaine	2.0	60	3	60-120	90-150
	Bupivacaine	0.5	15	3	90-240	240-300
	Tetracaine	0.5	15	3	90-240	240-300
	Cinchocaine	0.5	15	3	90-240	240-300
	Hypobaric					
	Bupivacaine	0.25	7.5-10	3-4	90-240	-
	Tetracaine	0.1-0.33	4-10	4-10	90-240	-
	Cinchocaine	0.067	3-7	5-10	90-240	-

* Although a dose range is given, the larger amounts are recommended to improve the quality of block and likelihood of success (p. 142)

** Duration of surgical anaesthesia

*** Epinephrine

**** See sections on vasoconstrictors p. 87 and 143. Epinephrine does not appear to prolong anaesthesia in the thoracic dermatomes. Some prolongation is observed in the lumbosacral regions. The prolongation shown here is merely an estimate of what may occur and is not necessarily experimentally determined.

Isobaric solutions of bupivacaine and lidocaine are not approved by the FDA for spinal anaesthesia. However, this use has been reported in numerous publications. Solutions used for spinal anaesthesia should **not** contain any preservatives or antioxidants such as methylparaben, sodium sulphite or sodium metabisulphite.

Adapted with permission, Lambert and Covino[72]

References

1. Kehlet H (1984) The stress response to anaesthesia and surgery: release mechanisms and modifying factors. Clin Anesth 1984;2:315

2. Svartling N, Lehtinen AM, Tarkkanen L (1986) The effect of anaesthesia on changes in blood pressure and plasma cortisol levels induced by cementation and methylmethacrylate. Acta Anaesthesiol Scand 30:247

3. Davis FM, Laurenson VG, Lewis J, Wells JE, Gillespie WJ (1987) Metabolic response to total hip arthroplasty under hypobaric subarachnoid or general anaesthesia. Br J Anaesth 59:725

4. Pflug AE, Halter JB (1981) Effect of spinal anesthesia on adrenergic tone and the neuroendocrine responses to surgical stress in humans. Anesthesiology 55:120

5. Oyama T, Matsuki A (1970) Effects of spinal anaesthesia on carbohydrate and fat metabolism in man. Br J Anaesth 42:723

6. Aitkenhead AR, Wishart HY, Brown DAP (1978) High spinal nerve block for large bowel anastomosis: a retrospective study. Br J Anaesth 50:177

7. Thorburn J, Louden JR, Vallance R (1980) Spinal and general anaesthesia in total hip replacement: frequency of deep vein thrombosis. Br J Anaesth 52:1117

8. McKenzie PJ, Wishart HY, Dewar MS, Gray I, Smith G (1980) Comparison of the effects of spinal anaesthesia and general anaesthesia on postoperative oxygenation and perioperative mortality. Br. J. Anaesth 52:49

9. McKenzie PJ, Wishart HY, Smith G (1984) Long term outcome after repair of fractured neck of femur. Br J Anaesth 56:581

10. Hedenstierna G, Löfström J (1985) Effect of anaesthesia on respiratory function after major lower extremity surgery. Acta Anaesthesiol Scand 29:55

11. McKenzie PJ, Wishart HY, Gray I, Smith G (1985) Effects of anaesthetic technique on deep vein thrombosis: a comparison of subarachnoid and general anaesthesia. Br J Anaesth 57:853

12. Cook PT, Davies MJ, Cronin KD, Moran P (1986) A prospective randomized trial comparing spinal anaesthesia using hyperbaric cinchocaine with general anaesthesia for lower limb vascular surgery. Anaesth Intens Care 14:373

13. Johnson A, Bengtsson M, Mertis H, Löfström JB (1986) Anesthesia for major hip surgery: a clinical study of spinal and general anesthesia in 244 patients. Reg Anaesth 11:83

14. Valentin N, Lomholt B, Jensen JS, Hejgaard N, Kreiner S (1986) Spinal or general anaesthesia for surgery of the fractured hip: a prospective study of mortality in 578 patients. Br J Anesth 58:284

15. Davis FM, McDermott E, Hickton C, Wells E, Heaton DC, Laurenson VG, Gillespie WJ, Foate J (1987) Influence of spinal and general anaesthesia on haemostasis during total hip arthoplasty. Br J Anaesth 59:561

16. Covino BG (1989) Rationale for spinal anesthesia. Int Anesth Clin 27:8

17. McGowan SW, Smith GFN (1980) Anaesthesia for transurethral prostactectomy: a comparison of spinal intradural analgesia with two methods of general anaesthesia. Anaesthesia 35:847

18. Modig J, Borg T, Karlström G, Maripuu E, Sahlstedt B (1983) Thromboembolism after total hip replacement. Role of epidural and general anesthesia. Anesth Analg 62:174

19. Foate JA, Horton H, Davis FM (1985) Lower limb blood flow during transurethral resection of the prostate under spinal or general anesthesia. Anaesth Intensive Care 13:383

20. McLaren AD, Stockwell MC, Reid VT (1978) Anaesthetic techniques for surgical correction of fractured neck of femur. Br J Anaesth 33:10

21. Davis FM, Laurenson VG (1981) Spinal anaesthesia or general anaesthesia for emergency hip surgery in elderly patients. Anaesth Intensive Care 9:352

22. Ward RJ, Bonica JJ, Freund FG, Akamatsu T, Danzinger F, Englesson S (1965) Epidural and subarachnoid anesthesia: cardiovascular and respiratory effects. JAMA 191:275

23. Valli H, Rosenberg PH (1985) Effects of three anaesthesia methods on haemodynamic responses connected with the use of thigh tourniquet in orthopaedic patients. Acta Anaesthesiol Scand 29:142

24. Baker AS, Ojemann RG, Swartz MN, Richardson EP (1975) Spinal epidural abscess. N Engl J of Med 293:463

25. Eng RHK, Seligman SJ (1981) Lumbar puncture-induced meningitis. JAMA 245:1456

26. Rao TKL, El-Etr AA (1981) Anticoagulation following placement of epidural and subarachnoid catheter. Anesthesiology 56:618

27. Allemann BH, Gerber H, Gruber UF (1983) Rückenmarksnahe Anaesthesie und subkutan verabreichtes low-dose Heparin-Dihydergot zur Thromboembolieprophylaxe. [Perispinal anesthesia and subcutaneous administration of low-dose heparin-dihydergot for prevention of thromboembolism]. Anaesthetist 32:80

28. Benson HT, Brunner EA, Vaisrub N (1984) Bleeding time and nerve blocks after aspirin. Reg Anesth 9:86

29. Horlocker TT, Wedel DJ, Offord KP (1990) Does preoperative antiplatelet therapy increase the risk of hemorrhagic complications associated with regional anesthesia? Anesth Analg 70:631

30. Dalen JE, Evans GL, Banas JS, Brooks HL, Paraskos JA (1969) Dexter L. The hemodynamic and respiratory effects of diazepam (Valium). Anesthesiology 30:259

31. Reves JG, Fragen RJ, Vinick HR, Greenblatt DJ (1985) Midazolam: pharmacology and uses. Anesthesiology 62:310

32. Griffiths HWC, Gilles J (1948) Thoraco-lumbar splanchnic-tectomy and sympathectomy: anesthetic procedure. Anaesthesia 3:134

33. Miller MI, Lorhan P (1955) Clinical evaluation of hypotensive spinal anesthesia. Anesthesiology 16:73

34. Scott DB (1991) Pelvic surgery. In: MacRae W, Wildsmith J eds. Induced hypotension. Amsterdam: Elsevier, 299

35. MacRae WR, Wildsmith JAW (1991) Induced hypotension. Amsterdam: Elsevier, 338

36. Caplan RA, Ward RJ, Posner K, Cheney FW (1988) Unexpected cardiac arrest during spinal anesthesia: a closed claims analysis of predisposing factors. Anesthesiology 68:5

37. Caplan RA, Posner KL, Ward RJ, Cheney FW (1990) Adverse respiratory events in anesthesia: a closed claims analysis. Anesthesiology 72:828

38. Tinker JH, Dull DL, Caplan RA, Ward RJ, Cheney FW (1989) Role of monitoring devices in prevention of anesthesia mishaps: a closed claims analysis. Anesthesiology 71:541

39. Cohen S, Daitch JS, Goldiner PL (1989) An alternative method for management of accidental dural puncture for labor and deliver (letter). Anesthesiology 70:164

40. Norris MC, Leighton BL (1990) Continuous spinal anesthesia after unintentional dural puncture in parturients. Reg Anesth 15:285

41. Russell IF (1983). Spinal anaesthesia for caesarean section. The use of 0.5% bupivacaine. Br J Anaesth 55:309

42. Hunt CO, Naulty JS, Bader AM, et al. (1989) Perioperative analgesia with subarachnoid fentanyl-bupivacaine for cesarean delivery. Anesthesiology 71:535

43 Scott DB (1968) Inferior vena caval occlusion in late pregnancy and its importance in anaesthesia. Br J Anaesth 40:120

44. Murray AM, Morgan M, Whitwam JG (1989) Crystalloid versus colloid for circulatory preload for epidural caesarean section. Anaesthesia 44:463

45. Robson S, Hunter S, Boys R, Dunlop W, Bryson M (1989) Changes in cardiac output during epidural anaesthesia for caeserean section. Anaesthesia 44:475

46. Datta S, Alper MH, Ostheimer GW, Weiss JB (1982) Method of ephedrine administration and nausea and hypotension during spinal anesthesia for cesarean section. Anesthesiology 56:68

47 Welborn LG, Rice LJ, Hannallah RS, Broadman LM, Ruttimann UE, Fink R (1990) Postoperative apnea in former preterm infants: prospective comparison of spinal and general anesthesia. Anesthesiology 72:838

48. Abajian JC, Mellish RW, Browne AF, Perkins FM, Lambert DH, Mazuzan JE (1984) Spinal anesthesia for surgery in the high risk infant. Anesth Analg 63:358

49. Rice LJ (1988) Regional anesthesia in pediatrics. In ASA 39th annual refresher course lectures and clinical update program. Illinois: American Society of Anesthesiologists 123

50. Saint-Maurice C (1990) Spinal block. In: Saint-Maurice C, Schulte-Steinberg 0 ed. Regional anesthesia in children. Fribourg, Switzerland: Mediglobe, 123

51. Parkinson SK, Little WL, Malley RA, Pecsok JL, Mueller JB, Whalen T (1990). Use of hyperbaric bupivacaine with epinephrine for spinal anesthesia in infants. Reg Anesth 15:86

52. Cousins MJ, Cherry DA, Gourlay GK (1988) Acute and chronic pain: use of spinal opiods. In: Cousins M, Bridenbaugh P ed. Neural blockade. Philadelphia: JB Lippincott, Co., 1006

53. Coombs DW, Maurer LH, Saunders RL, Gaylor M (1984) Outcomes and complications of intraspinal narcotic analgesia for cancer pain control. J Clin Oncol 2:1414

54. Penn RD, Paice JA, Gottschalk W, Ivankovich AD (1984) Cancer pain relief using chronic morphine infusion. Early experience with a programmable implanted drug pump. J Neurosurg 61:302

55. Bonica JJ, Buckley FP, Moricca G, Murphy TM (1990) Neurolytic blockage and hypophysectomy. In: Bonica J ed. The management of pain. Philadelphia: Lea & Febiger, 1991

56. Rosomoff HL, Papo I, Loeser JD, Bonica JJ (1990) Neurosurgical operations on the spinal cord. In: Bonica J ed. The management of pain. Philadelphia: Lea & Febiger, 2067

57. Greene NM (1985) Distribution of local anesthetic solutions within the subarachnoid space. Anesth Analg 64:715

58. Lambert DH (1989) Factors influencing spinal anesthesia. Int Anesthesiol Clin 27:13

59. Norris MC (1988) Height, weight, and the spread of subarachnoid hyperbaric bupivacaine in the term parturient. Anesth Analg 67:555

60. Sheskey MC, Rocco AG, Bizzarri-Schmid M, Francis DM, Edström H, Covino BG (1983) A dose-response study of bupivacaine for spinal anesthesia. Anesth Analg 62:931

61. Wildsmith JA, McClure JH, Brown DT, Scott DB (1981) Effect of posture on the spread of isobaric and hyperbaric amethocaine. Br J Anaesth 53:273

62. Brown DT, Wildsmith JA, Covino BG, Scott DB (1980) Effects of baricity on spinal anaesthesia with amethocaine. Br J Anaesth 52:589

63. Tuominen M, Taivainen T, Rosenberg PH (1989) Spread of spinal anesthesia with plain bupivacaine: influence of the vertebral interspace used for injection. BR J Anaesth 62:358

64. Collins JG, Kitahata LM, Matsumoto M (1984) Spinally administered epinephrine suppresses noxiously evoked activity of WDR neurons in the dorsal horn of the spinal cord. Anesthesiology 60:269

65 Vaida GT, Moss P, Capan LM, Turndoff H (1986) Prolongation of lidocaine spinal anesthesia with phenylephrine. Anesth Analg 65:781

66. Lawrence VS, Rich CR, Magitzky L, Lee JH (1984) Spinal anesthesia with isobaric lidocaine 2% and the effect of phenylephrine. Reg Anesth 9:17

67. Racle JP, Benkhadra A, Poy JY, Gleizal B (1987) Effects of increasing amounts of epinephrine during isobaric spinal anesthesia in elderly patients. Anesth Analg 66:882

68. Meagher RP, Moore DC, DeVries JC (1966) Phenylephrine: the most effective potentiator of tetracaine spinal anesthesia. Anesth Analg 45:134

69. Chambers WA, Littlewood DG, Logan MR, Scott DB (1982) Effect of added epineprine on spinal anesthesia with lidocaine. Anesth Analg 60:417

70. Chambers WA, Littlewood DG, Scott DB (1982) Spinal anesthesia with hyperbaric bupivacaine: effect of added vasoconstrictors. Anesth Analg 61:49

71. Armstrong IR, Littlewood DG, Chambers WA (1983) Spinal anesthesia with tetracaine - effect of added vasoconstrictors. Anesth Analg 62:793

72. Lambert DH, Covino BG (1987) Hyperbaric, hypobaric and isobaric spinal anesthesia. Res Staff Phys 33:79

Chapter 6

Complications of spinal anaesthesia

Treatment of hypotension during spinal anaesthesia depends on proper assessment of the cause. If the hypotension is sudden and accompanied by bradycardia and nausea, then vasovagal syncope should be suspected. **Atropine is often given in this situation but it is much less effective than a vasopressor** (see p. 62).[20]

The low pressure is more usually due to decreased peripheral resistance and cardiac output. This is the cause of hypotension due to sympathetic blockade or when a light general anaesthetic has been added. It is relatively benign and forms the basis of induced hypotension with high spinal blockade (see p. 134). As such it can be employed to reduce blood loss in operations where this is considered beneficial.[21]

The pulse rate will usually be in the normal range (60-80 beats/min) though young patients may develop a mild tachycardia (80-120 beats/min). If the block is high enough to affect the cardiac accelerator fibres, then a mild bradycardia (50-60 beats/min) will result.

Vasopressor agents (Table 6.1)
These may be pure α-adrenoceptor stimulators, e.g. phenylephrine, or combined α- and β-stimulators, e.g. ephedrine. Methoxamine, which is primarily an α-stimulator, causes reversal of the hypotension but produces bradycardia, with a reduction in cardiac output. This may or may not improve the balance between oxygen supply and demand of the myocardium in patients with coronary artery disease.[22,23] Methoxamine should be avoided in treating hypotension during Caesarean section, however, as it has been shown to decrease uterine blood flow.[24,25] All of these agents are very rapid in their effect and when given intravenously care should be taken to avoid hypertension. If given intramuscularly their action is slower and more prolonged. Thus combined IV and IM injection will raise the pressure quickly and maintain it for a longer time. Short- acting drugs such as phenylephrine or norepinephrine given by infusion have the advantages of rapid and accurate control of the arterial pressure, and a short duration of effect when stopped.

Dihydroergotamine, which causes vasoconstriction of capacitance vessels, has been used to increase venous return in spinal and epidural anaesthesia.[26]

Table 6.1. The drugs used for treating hypotension.

Drug	Administration	Effects
Ephedrine	Repeated IV boluses (5-10 mg) or IV infusion (50 mg in 500 mL dextrose, 20-50 mL initially, then according to effect)	α and β activity
Phenylephrine	IV infusion (20 mg in 500 mL dextrose, 1-2ml initially, then according to effect)	α activity only
Methoxamine	Repeated IV boluses (3-5 mg)	α activity Decreases heart rate and cardiac output Decreases uterine blood flow in late pregnancy
Dihydroergotamine	Repeated IV boluses 0.5 mg	Venoconstriction and weak arterial constriction

Posture

All patients with hypotension should be tilted head down to avoid pooling of blood in the legs. A useful rise in pressure due to increased cardiac output usually follows this simple manoeuvre.[7] If the hypotension is thought to be due to inferior vena caval occlusion, then this must be relieved by an appropriate change of posture.[27]

Intravenous fluids

The use of fluids to increase circulating blood volume will counteract hypotension even in patients not clinically hypovolaemic. Crystalloids are just as effective as colloids in the short term and can be eliminated quickly if renal function is adequate.[17] If treatment of the hypotension is not urgent, rapid infusion (250-500 mL of crystalloid in 5-10 min) is usually effective. In patients with normal hydration, it is seldom necessary to give more that 1-1.5 L of fluid during the 1-3 h of the block.

Only vasopressors are capable of reversing the prime cause of this type of hypotension, i.e. the decrease in peripheral resistance. Posture and fluids work by increasing cardiac output. The effect of fluids therefore is less pronounced and less rapid than that of vasopressors.

Cardiac arrest

This is a rare complication of spinal block[28] but may result from severe hypotension and consequent myocardial ischaemia. The hypotension may be the result of syncope[8] or a high block in a severely hypovolaemic patient. In such cases the patient should respond to urgent cardiopulmonary resuscitation together with vasopressors (including epinephrine) and fluids as appropriate.[28]

Respiratory failure

This may occur if a particularly high block leads to paralysis of the muscles of respiration. Paralysis of the lower intercostal muscles is quite common but does not affect normal quiet respiration.[29] Even with all the intercostal muscles paralysed, the diaphragm still provides adequate ventilation in most patients.[29] If the patient complains of dyspnoea, however, assisted or controlled respiration may be required. If significant respiratory depression is present, it is best to induce general anaesthesia, intubate the trachea and ventilate the patient.

Failed spinal blockade

Sometimes a spinal blockade fails to develop in spite of an apparently successful lumbar puncture. In most cases the local anaesthetic was not in fact injected into the subarachnoid space. The anaesthesiologist should always have a contingency plan for a failed block. The alternatives are either to repeat the spinal anaesthesia or to convert to a general anaesthetic.

High or total spinal blockade

This is an unusual complication if the recommended doses of local anaesthetic drugs are used. However, if for any reason the block ascends too high, unconsciousness can occur and the muscles of respiration, including the diaphragm, may be paralysed, in which case artificial ventilation becomes mandatory. In spite of this alarming clinical picture, the patient can be safely managed with respiratory and circulatory support until the local anaesthetic effects have worn off.

Postdural puncture headache

This is the most common postoperative complication of spinal anaesthesia. The cause of the headache is the loss of CSF from the subarachnoid to the epidural space through the needle hole in the dura mater. Decreased brain buoyancy owing to low intracranial pressure causes traction on the structures supporting the brain and on the cranial nerves themselves. The cranial nerves mediating the headache are thought to be the trigeminal, the glossopharyngeal and the vagus, but traction on the trochlear and the abducent can cause paralysis of the ocular muscles. The headache is often accompanied by neck pain and stiffness, presumably mediated by the upper cervical nerves.

The amount of CSF escaping through the dura depends upon the size and shape of the hole and the pressure difference between the subarachnoid and epidural spaces. Spinal CSF pressure is much greater in the upright posture than when lying down, and explains the relationship between posture and the headache. The headache, which is often severe, is maximal when upright and quickly relieved by lying down. Postdural puncture headache (PDPH) must be differentiated from other types of headache such as migraine or that due to meningitis.

Needle size and shape (p. 106)

The size of the dural hole relates to the outside diameter of the spinal needle and the trend towards using fine needles is because of the lower incidence of headache associated with them. The shape of the needle tip is also important. Cutting fewer fibres of the dura mater reduces the size of the hole. Thus tips which stretch the dural fibres rather than cut them, e.g. the pencil point needles, reduce the incidence of PDPH. Other needles have a cutting edge only on part of the tip, creating an initial small "cut" through which the rest of the needle stretches the fibres as it passes into the subarachnoid space.

Dura mater

While the dura is made of tough fibrous tissue its thickness varies considerably even in the same individual. Its fibres generally run longitudinally, but there are also transverse fibres.[30] The orientation of the needle bevel during lumbar puncture is important, as the needle tip cuts fewer longitudinal fibres if the bevel is oriented longitudinally rather than transversely (see p. 20 and p. 112).[31]

The hole left by a needle in the dura mater resembles an opened tin can rather than a neat punched out hole. The resulting flap may fall back into place, virtually sealing the hole.

The arachnoid mater is closely applied to the dura but is not attached to it. For CSF to leak, the hole in the dura must be very close to the hole in the arachnoid. An angled approach to the subarachnoid space is associated with a lower incidence of headache.[32]

The great number of factors affecting the amount of CSF leakage explains the wide variation in the quoted incidence of PDPH even using the same needle size. Patients who have had a dural puncture with a 16 or 18 gauge needle may have no headache, while others develop a headache after puncture with a 29 gauge needle.

Age

Younger patients are more likely to develop PDPH though the reasons for this are not clear.[33,34]

Sex

Females are said to be more liable to PDPH but this may be related to the fact that many women receive spinal anaesthesia in obstetrics, while the most common indication in men is urology, i.e. the sexes differ in regard to their age when receiving a spinal.

Clinical features

PDPH can appear as late as 5 days after lumbar puncture, although it usually occurs within a few hours of resuming the upright posture and ambulation. It can be frontal or occipital or both and frequently affects the neck as well. It is clearly related to posture. In severe cases it can cause mental depression and debilitation. Without treatment PDPH usually lasts 3-7 days, but can last much longer. Severe cases can be associated with abducent or trochlear nerve palsies leading to strabismus and double vision. Hearing loss has also been reported during PDPH.

Cranial subdural haematoma is a rare but recognized complication of the prolonged reduction in CSF pressure.[35]

Prophylaxis

The incidence of PDPH may be reduced by:

1. The use of small diameter lumbar puncture needles.[33,34,36]

2. The use of needle points designed to produce minimal damage to dural fibres rather than cut them..[36]

3. Aligning the needle bevel longitudinally, so as to separate the longitudinal dural fibres.[31]

4. The use of the paramedian approach.[37]

5. Avoiding multiple puncture holes in the dura mater.

6. Ensuring that the patient does not become dehydrated.

Bed rest and avoiding the upright position will delay but not prevent the onset of PDPH. Keeping patients flat in bed for 24 h after a spinal anaesthetic does not reduce the incidence of PDPH.[38,39]

Treatment

If the headache is not severe and not interfering with normal activity, simple methods of treatment are recommended, e.g. bed rest, analgesics or caffeine,[40-42] which has a cerebral vasoconstrictor effect.

If the PDPH is severe and incapacitating it is advisable to proceed as soon as possible to a "blood patch". This involves the injection of 10-15 mL of homologous blood into the epidural space.[43] This increases the CSF pressure considerably, while decreasing the amount of CSF leakage. Unlike saline and other fluids, blood is not quickly removed from the epidural space. Particular care with aseptic precautions is necessary. The success rate with epidural blood patch is high (>90%) although it must occasionally be repeated. Very few complications have been reported.

Backache

Backache after spinal anaesthesia is relatively infrequent. This may relate to the fact that backache is usually not severe and postoperative analgesia for surgical pain may conceal the lesser pain of backache.

A small haematoma, ligamentous injury, reflex muscle spasm, etc. produced by the lumbar puncture may be responsible for the backache. Positioning during operation is another factor often considered to cause backache. Profound muscle relaxation coupled with the lithotomy position can result in lumbar ligamentous strain during spinal anaesthesia.[44]

Although the incidence of backache in hospitalized patients is low, there is a 30-50% incidence of mild backache in outpatients.[45] In one study, only 3% of outpatients graded the backache as severe and 12% as moderate.[46] However, no careful comparison of backache in hospitalized versus ambulatory patients has been conducted. Furthermore, the mild nature of the backache should not be a contraindication to the use of spinal anaesthesia in ambulatory patients.[44]

When severe backache occurs after spinal anaesthesia, major neurological injury and in particular a space occupying lesion (vide infra) must be ruled out. Otherwise, reassurance, rest, local application of heat and analgesics rectify the problem. Fortunately, backache after spinal anaesthesia is transient, resolving in 48 h or so with conservative therapy. Occasionally, paraspinous muscle spasm is the cause, and trigger point injection with a local anaesthetic, or anti-inflammatory agents given with a benzodiazepine are useful.[44]

Neurological complications

The fear of permanent neurological damage following spinal anaesthesia was a considerable disincentive to the use of spinal anaesthesia for many years. It cannot be denied that cases do occur, albeit very rarely, and the issue must be addressed.

It is important to understand the different pathological processes that can cause neurological damage and to diagnose that which is involved in an individual case. These include:

Pre-existing disease

There are examples in the literature of patients relating their first symptoms of neurological disease to spinal anaesthesia,[47] e.g. in malignant disease of the spine or multiple sclerosis.[48] Spinal anaesthesia is not involved in the causation, and is most unlikely to adversely affect such conditions. Careful history taking (including the testimony of relatives) may reveal minor but important symptoms of unsuspected neurological conditions.

Direct trauma to a spinal nerve or the spinal cord

As elsewhere in the body, the insertion of a needle into a nerve in the cauda equina and, more importantly, the injection of fluid into that nerve, can cause disruption of nerve fibres. With an intraneural injection, the local anaesthetic can spread along the nerve root to the spinal cord and damage the cell bodies.[49] The result is pain during the needle insertion and/or the injection, followed by paraesthesia or hypoalgesia in the distribution of the nerve. Sometimes there is also some motor weakness. This type of injury fortunately resolves after a few weeks, but occasionally it lasts much longer. If the spinal cord itself is injured, the end result may be much more serious, but use of the lower lumbar intervertebral spaces for lumbar puncture should prevent its occurrence.

Cauda equina syndrome

Cauda equina syndrome occurs when the cauda equina is injured or compressed. Signs and symptoms are confined to areas innervated by the lumbar and sacral nerves. These include autonomic dysfunction, alterations in evacuation of bladder and bowel, abnormal sweating and temperature control, and motor weakness, as well as altered pinprick, temperature and position sensation in the affected dermatomes.[49]

The causes of cauda equina syndrome are trauma or toxicity. When neither traumatic puncture nor intraneural injection occurred, the assumption is that a toxic substance was injected into the CSF. This could be a contaminant such as a detergent or antiseptic,[50] a preservative[3] or an excessive amount of local anaesthetic.[51-53]

There have been recent reports of cauda equina syndrome after continous spinal anaesthesia with small-bore catheters (see p. 123).[51-53] The mechanism for the injury is hypothesized to be poor dilution of the local anaesthetic in the CSF, such that the thinly sheathed cauda equina nerves are directly exposed to toxic concentrations of the local anaesthetic, which might develop if the local anaesthetic (when injected slowly through a long, high resistance microcatheter) displaces the CSF instead of being diluted by thoroughly mixing with the CSF, as is the case when it is injected quickly through a spinal needle. In this regard, directly exposing isolated desheated nerves (believed to be similar to cauda equina nerves) to concentrations of the local anaesthetics commonly used for spinal anaesthesia, shows that they are neurotoxic, *per se*.[54] The hypertonic dextrose used to make spinal anaesthetic solutions hyperbaric may also be toxic to the cauda equina. However, the isolated nerve studies indicate that this is probably not the case.[54]

Spinal cord infarction

The blood supply to the lower spinal cord is somewhat tenuous, being mainly through the artery of Adamkiewicz (see p. 25). Failure of this blood supply, the anterior spinal artery syndrome, will cause an infarction of the spinal cord leading to a rapid onset of painless paraplegia. Profound hypotension has been implicated, particularly in the presence of atherosclerosis, and indeed spontaneous cases are well recognized in arteriosclerotic patients. The addition of vasoconstrictors to the injected local anaesthetic has been suggested as a cause, but there is little evidence for it. It is important to remember that spinal cord infarction can be due to other causes such as vascular anomalies, the application of high aortic clamps or surgical retraction involving the aorta.[55]

Space occupying lesions of the spinal canal

Because these conditions are often treatable if the diagnosis is made without delay, it is important to be aware of the clinical picture and to initiate urgent investigations. Compression of the cord or the cauda equina causes backache (often severe) and loss of function in the spinal nerves below the level of compression, with areflexia, muscle weakness and sensory loss. These features can be affected by any remaining spinal anaesthesia, but patients complaining of severe backache should be examined quickly and thoroughly. The most common conditions are epidural haematoma, epidural abscess and unsuspected malignant disease of the spine.

Meningitis

The introduction of bacteria into the subarachnoid space is unlikely if adherence to good clinical practice is maintained. Aseptic meningitis, presumably due to the injection of chemical irritants, has been described (see p. 156), but should not occur with disposable equipment and the appropriate amount of pure local anaesthetic solutions.

Adhesive arachnoiditis

This is probably the most common serious neurological complication of spinal anaesthesia. The cause is invariably the injection of an irritant substance into the subarachnoid space.[49] Such an injection is frequently painful at the time. The onset and progress of the arachnoiditis is also painful but may be slow, taking hours or days to develop fully. The careful checking of ampoules, syringes, etc., before the injection is important, but less obvious problems can arise, e.g. the incomplete removal of detergent if reusable glass syringes are employed.[50] The habit of keeping spinal ampoules in antiseptic has long disappeared in most countries, but may still be used in the Third World, and should be abandoned.

Summary

Provided the above complications are well understood, they can usually be avoided or dealt with safely and expeditiously. There is no substitute for meticulous attention to detail. It was shown many years ago by Dripps and Vandam that large numbers of spinal anaesthetics could be performed without serious morbidity and with important advantages to the patients.[56]

References

1. Reisner LS, Hochman BN, Plumer MH (1980) Persistent neurologic deficit and adhesive arachnoiditis following intrathecal 2-chloroprocaine injection. Aneth Analg 59:452

2. Ravindran RS, Bond VK, Tasch MD, Gupta CD, Luerssen TG (1980) Prolonged neural blockade following regional analgesia with 2-chloroprocaine. Anesth Analg 59:447

3. Gissen AJ, Datta S, Lambert D (1984) The chloroprocaine controversy. II. Is chloroprocaine neurotoxic? Reg Anesth 9:135

4. Rigler ML, Drasner K, Krejcie TC, Yelich SJ, Scholnick FT, DeFontes J, Bohner D (1991) Cauda Equina Syndrome after continuous spinal anesthesia. Anesth Analg 72:275

5. Greene NM (1981) Physiology of spinal anesthesia. (3rd ed.). Baltimore: Williams & Wilkins, 116

6. Ward RJ, Bonica JJ, Freund FG, Akamatsu T, Danzinger F, Englesson S (1965) Epidural and subarachnoid anesthesia: cardiovascular and respiratory effects. JAMA 191 :275

7. Greene NM (1981) Preganglionic sympathetic blockade in man: a study of spinal anesthesia. Acta Anaesth Scand 25:463

8. Mackey DC, Carpenter RL, Thompson GE, Brown DL, Bodily MN (1989) Bradycardia and asystole during spinal anesthesia: a report of three cases without morbidity. Anesthesiology 70:866

9. Stephen GW, Lees MM, Scott DB (1969) Cardiovascular effects of epidural block combined with general anesthesia. Br J Anaesth 41:933

10. Griffiths HWC, Gilles J (1948) Thoraco-lumbar splanchnicectomy and sympathectomy: anesthetic procedure. Anaesthesia 3:134

11. Miller MI, Lorhan P (1955). Clinical evaluation of hypotensive spinal anesthesia. Anesthesiology 16:73

12. Scott DB (1982) Cardiovascular effects of lumbar epidural and spinal anesthesia. Reg Anesth [Suppl] 7:S21

13. Hackel DB, Sancetta SM, Kleinerman L (1956) Effect of hypotension due to spinal anesthesia on coronary blood flow and myocardial metabolism in man. Circulation 13:92

14. Sivarajan M, Armory DW, Lindbloom LE, Schwettman RS (1975) Systemic and regional blood-flow changes during spinal anesthesia in the Rhesus monkey. Anesthesiology 43:78

15. Greene NM (1981) Physiology of spinal anesthesia (3 ed.). Baltimore: Williams & Wilkins, 111

16. Wollman SB, Marks GF (1968) Acute hydration for prevention of hypotension of spinal anesthesia in parturients. Anesthesiology 29:374

17. Murray AM, Morgan M, Whitwam JG (1989) Crystalloid versus colloid for circulatory preload for epidural caesarean section. Anaesthesia 44:463

18. Robson S, Hunter S, Boys R, Dunlop W, Bryson M (1989) Changes in cardiac output during epidural anaesthesia for caesarean section. Anaesthesia 44:475

19. Dripps RD, Eckenhoff JE, Vandam LD (1977) Arterial hypotension during anesthesia. In: Introduction to anesthesia. The principles of safe practice. Philadelphia: W.B. Saunders Co., 414

20. Ward RJ, Kennedy W, Bonica JJ, Martin WE, Tolas AG, Akamatsu T (1966) Experimental evaluation of atropine and vasopressors for the treatment of hypotension of high subarachnoid anesthesia. Anesth Analg 45:621

21. Scott DB (1991) Pelvic surgery. In: MacRae W, Wildsmith J ed. Induced hypotension. Amsterdam: Elsevier, 299

22. Li T-H, Shimosato S, Etsten BE (1965) Methoxamine and cardiac output in non-anesthetized man and during spinal anesthesia. Anesthesiology 26:21

23. Smith NT, Corbascio AN (1970) The use and misuse of pressor agents. Anesthesiology 33:58

24. Eng M, Berges PU, Ueland K, Bonica JJ, Parer JT (1971) The effects of methoxamine and ephedrine in normotensive pregnant primates. Anesthesiology 35:354

25. Shnider SM, DeLorimier AA, Asling JH, Morishima HO (1970) Vasopressors in obstetrics. II. Fetal hazards of methoxamine administration during obstetric spinal anesthesia. Am J Obstet Gynecol 106:680-

26. Mattila M, Hannonen P, Puttonen E, Lappalainen S (1985) Dihydroergotamine in the prevention of hypotension associated with extradural anaesthesia. Br J Anaesth 57:976

27. Marx GF (1969) Supine hypotension syndrome during cesarean section. JAMA 207:1903

28. Caplan RA, Ward RJ, Posner K, Cheney FW (1988) Unexpected cardiac arrest during spinal anesthesia: a closed claims analysis of predisposing factors. Anesthesiology 68:5

29.Steinbrook RA (1989) Respiratory effects of spinal anesthesia. Int Anesthesiol Clin 27:40

30. Fink BR, Walker S (1989) Orientation of fibers in human dorsal lumbar dura in relation to lumbar puncture. Anesth Analg 69:768

31. Mihic DN (1985) Postspinal headache and relationship of needle bevel to longitudinal dural fibers. Reg Anesth 10:76

32. Hatfalvi BI (1977) The dynamics of post-spinal headache. Headache 17:64

33. Vandam LD, Dripps RD (1956) Long-term follow-up of patients who received 10,098 spinal anesthetics. III. Syndrome of decreased intracranial pressure (headache and ocular and auditory difficulties). JAMA 161:586

34. Gielen M (1989) Post dural puncture headache (PDPH). Reg Anesth 14:101

35. Macon ME, Armstrong L, Brown EM (1990) Subdural haemtoma following spinal anesthesia. Anesthesiology 72:380

36. Hurley RJ, Lambert DH, Hirtwig L, Datta S (1992) Post dural puncture headache in the obstetric patient: spinal versus epidural anesthesia. Anesthesiology 77:A1018

37. Ready LB, Cuplin S, Haschke RH, Nessly M (1989) Spinal needle determinants of rate of transdural fluid leak. Anesth Analg 69:457

38. Carbaat PAT, van Crevel H (1981) Lumbar puncture headache: controlled study of the preventive effect of 24 hours' bed rest. Lancet 2(8256):1133

39. Thomberry EA, Thomas TA (1988) Posture and post-spinal headache. A controlled trial in 80 obstetric patients. Br J Anaesth 60:195

40. Sechzer PH, Abel L (1978) Post-spinal anesthesia headache treated with caffeine. Evaluation with demand method. Part I. Curr Ther Res 24:307

41. Jarvis AP (1986) Intravenous caffeine for post-dural puncture headache. Reg Anesth 11:42

42. Camann WR, Murray RS, Mushlin PS, Lambert DH (1990) Effects of oral caffeine on postdural puncture headache: a double-blind, placebo controlled trial. Anesth Analg 70:181

43. Szeinfeld M, Ihmeidan IH, Moser MM, Machado R, Klose KJ, Serafini AN (1986) Epidural blood patch: evaluation of the volume and spread of blood injected into the epidural space. Anesthesiology 64:820

44. Lambert DH (1989) Complications of spinal anesthesia. Int Anesthesiol Clin 27:51

45. Flaatten H, Raeder J (1985) Spinal anesthesia for outpatient surgery. Anaesthesia 40:1108

46. Perz RR, Johnson DL, Shinozaki T (1988) Spinal anesthesia for outpatient surgery. Anesth Analg 67:S168

47. Vandam LD, Dripps RD (1956) Exacerbation of pre-existing neurologic disease after spinal anesthesia. N Engl J Med 255:843

48. Levesque P, Marsepoil T, Ho P, Venutolo F, Lesouef JM (1988) Sclerose en plaques revelee par une rachianesthesie [Multiple sclerosis disclosed by spinal anesthesia]. Ann Fr Anesth Reanim 7:68

49. Vandam LD (1986) Neurologic sequelae of spinal and epidural anesthesia. Int Anesthesiol Clin 24:231

50. Garfield JM, Andriole GL, Vetto JT, Richie JP (1986) Prolonged diabetes insipidus subsequent to an episode of chemical meningitis. Anesthesiology 64:253

51. Rigler ML, Drasner K, Krejcie TC, Yelich SJ, Scholnick FT, DeFontes J, Bohner D (1991) Cauda Equina Syndrome after continuous spinal anesthesia. Anesth Analg 72:275

52. Lambert DH, Hurley RJ (1991) Cauda equina syndrome and continuous spinal anesthesia. Anesth Analg 72:817

53. Schell R, Brauer F, Cole D, Il RA (1991) Persistent sacral nerve root deficits after continuous spinal anesthesia. Can J Anaesth 38:908

54. Lambert DH, Lambert LA, Strichartz GS (1992) Potential neurotoxicity of lidocaine solutions used for spinal anesthesia. Anesthesiology 77: A898

55. de-Mol B, Hamerlijnck R, Geest RD, Vermeulen FE (1989) Assessment of risk factors for spinal cord ischemia in surgery of thoracoabdominal aneurysms without use of adjuncts. Eur J Cardiothor Surg 3:449

56. Vandam LD, Dripps RD (1955) A long-term follow-up of 10,098 spinal anesthetics II. Incidence and analysis of minor neurologic defects. Surgery 38:463

57. Bouchard P, Caillet JB, Monnet F, Banssillon V (1984) Rachianesthesia et sclerose en plaque [Spinal anesthesia and multiple sclerosis]. Ann Fr Anaesth Reanim 3:194

Drug nomenclature

Throughout this book we have used the World Health Organization's International Non-proprietary Name (I.N.N.) convention. The alternative names of the various drugs, whether proprietary or generic, are given in this table.

I.N.N.	Other
Local anaesthetics	
Bupivacaine	Marcaine, Sensorcaine, Carbostesin
Chloroprocaine	2-chloroprocaine, Nesacaine
Cinchocaine	Dibucaine, Nupercaine
Etidocaine	Duranest
Lidocaine	Lignocaine, Xylocaine
Mepivacaine	Carbocaine
Prilocaine	Citanest
Procaine	Novocaine
Tetracaine	Amethocaine, Anethaine, Pontocaine, Pantocaine
Vasopressors & sympathomimetics	
Epinephrine	Adrenaline
Ephedrine	-
Methoxamine	Vasoxine, Vasoxyl
Phenylephrine	Neo-Synephrine
Opioids	
Fentanyl	Sublimaze
Hydromorphone	Dilaudid
Methadone	Amidone, Phenodone, Physeptone, Dolophine
Morphine	-
Naloxone	Narcan
Pethidine	Meperidine, Demerol, Dolantin
Sufentanil	Sufenta
Other drugs	
Chlormethiazole	Heminevrin, Hemineurin
Diazepam	Valium
Midazolam	Hypnovel
Temazepam	Normison, Euhypnos
Thiopental	Pentothal, Thiopentone

Index